EUSTACE MULLINS

MURDER BY INJECTION

THE STORY OF THE MEDICAL CONSPIRACY AGAINST AMERICA

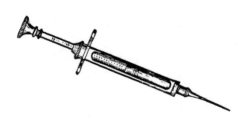

OMNIA VERITAS

EUSTACE CLARENCE MULLINS

(1923-2010)

MURDER BY INJECTION

THE STORY OF THE MEDICAL CONSPIRACY AGAINST AMERICA

1988

Published by

OMNIA VERITAS LTD

ℴMNIA VERITAS

www.omnia-veritas.com

For

BLAIR

in appreciation of your unequalled
dedication to American ideals

FOREWORD

The present work, the result of some forty years of investigative research, is a logical progression from my previous books: the expose of the international control of monetary issue and banking practices in the United States; a later work revealing the secret network of organizations through which these alien forces wield political power—the secret committees, foundations, and political parties through which their hidden plans are implemented; and now; to the most vital issue of all, the manner in which these depredations affect the daily lives and health of American citizens. Despite the great power of the hidden rulers, I found that only one group has the power to issue life or death sentences to any American—our nation's physicians.

I discovered that these physicians, despite their great power, were themselves subjected to very strict controls over every aspect of their professional lives. These controls, surprisingly enough, were not wielded by any state or federal agency, although almost every other aspect of American life is now under the absolute control of the bureaucracy. The physicians have their own autocracy, a private trade association, the American Medical Association. This group, which is headquartered in Chicago, Illinois, had gradually built up its power until it assumed total control over medical schools and the accreditation of physicians.

The trail of these manipulators led me straight to the same lairs of the international conspirators whom I had exposed in previous books. I knew that they had already looted America, reduced its military power to a dangerously low level, and imposed bureaucratic controls on every

American. I now discovered that their conspiracies also directly affected the health of every American.

This conspiracy has resulted in a documented decline in the health of our citizens. We now rank far down the list of civilized nations in infant mortality and other significant medical statistics. I was able to document the shocking record of these cold-blooded tycoons who not only plan and carry out famines, economic depressions, revolutions and wars, but who also find their greatest profits in their manipulations of our medical care. The cynicism and malice of these conspirators is something beyond the imagination of most Americans. They deliberately mulct our people of millions of dollars each year through "charitable" organizations and then use these same organizations as key groups to bolster their Medical Monopoly. Fear and intimidation are the basic techniques by which the conspirators maintain their control over all aspects of our health care, as they ruthlessly crush any competitor who challenges their profits. As in other aspects of their "behavioural control" over the American people, their most constantly used weapon against us is their employment of federal agents and federal agencies to carry out their intrigues. The proof of this operation may be the most disturbing revelation of my work.

Eustace Mullins
February 22, 1988

Acknowledgement:

I am grateful to the staff of the Library of Congress in Washington, D.C. for their courtesy and cooperation in the preparation of this work.

CHAPTER 1

THE MEDICAL MONOPOLY

The practice of medicine may not be the world's oldest profession, but it is often seen to be operating on much the same principles. Not only does the client wonder if he is getting what he is paying for, but in many instances, he is dismayed to find that he has actually gotten something he had not bargained for. An examination of the record shows that the actual methods of medical practice have not changed that much through the eons. The recently discovered Ebers papyrus shows that as early as 1600 B.C., more than nine hundred prescriptions were available to the physician, including opium as a pain-killing drug. As late as 1700, commonly used medications included cathartics such as senna, aloe, figs and castor oil. Intestinal worms were treated by aspidium roots (the male fern), pomegranate bark, or wormseed oil. In the East this was obtained from the flowers of santonin; in the Western Hemisphere it was pressed from the fruit and leaves of chenopodium.

Analgesics or pain relievers were alcohol, hyoscyamus leaves, and opium. Hyoscyamus contains scopolamine, used to induce "twilight sleep" in modern medicine. In the sixteenth century, Arabs used colchicum, a saffron derivative, for rheumatic pains and gout. Cinchona bark, the source of quinine, was used to treat malaria; chaulmoogra oil was used for leprosy, and ipecac for amoebic dysentery. Burned sponge at one time was used as a treatment for goiter; its content of iodine provided the cure. Midwives used ergot to contract the uterus. Some two hundred years ago, the era of modern medicine was ushered in by Sir Humphry Davy's discovery of the anaesthetic properties of nitrous oxide. Michael Faraday discovered ether, and Wilhelm Surtner isolated morphine from opium.

Until the late nineteenth century, doctors practiced as free lance agents, which meant that they assumed all the risks of their decisions. The poor rarely encountered a doctor, as medical ministrations were generally confined to the rich and powerful.

Curing a monarch could bring great rewards but failing to cure him could be a fatal mistake. Perhaps it was the awareness of the personal risks of this profession which gave rise to the plan for monopoly, to level out the risks and rewards among a chosen few. The attempts to build up this medical monopoly have now created a modern plague, while the resolve to maintain this monopoly has cost the public dearly in money and suffering.

Almost five centuries ago, one of the first attempts to set up this monopoly took place in England. The Act of 1511, signed into law by King Henry the Eighth, in England, made it an offence to practice physic or surgery without the approval of a panel of "experts." This Act was formalized in 1518 with the founding of the Royal College of Physicians. In 1540, barbers and surgeons were granted similar powers, when the King granted approval of their company. They immediately launched a campaign to eliminate the unauthorized practitioners who had served the poor. Apparently there is nothing new under the sun, as much the same campaign has long been underway in the United States. This harassment of doctors who served the poor caused such widespread suffering in England that King Henry the 8th was forced to enact the Quacks Charter in 1542. This Charter exempted the "unauthorized practitioners" and allowed them to continue their ministrations. No such charter has ever been granted in the United States, where a "quack" is not only an unauthorized practitioner, that is, one who has not been "approved" by the American Medical Association or one of the government agencies under its control, but he is also subject to immediate arrest. It is interesting that the chartering of quacks is not one of the features of English life which was passed on to its American colony.

In 1617, the Society of Apothecaries was formed in England. In 1832, the British Medical Association was chartered; this became the impetus for the forming of a similar association, the American Medical Association, in the United States. From its earliest inception, the American Medical Association has had one principal objective, attaining and defending a total monopoly of the practice of medicine in the United States. From its outset, the AMA made allopathy the basis of its practice. Allopathy was a type of medicine whose practitioners had received training in a recognized academic school of medicine, and who relied heavily on surgical procedures and the use of medications. The leaders of this brand of medicine had been trained in Germany. They were dedicated to the frequent use of bleeding and heavy doses of drugs. They were inimical to any form of medicine which had not proceeded from the academies and which did not follow standardized or orthodox procedures.

Allopathy set up an intense rivalry with the prevalent nineteenth school of medicine, the practice of homeopathy. This school was the creation of a doctor named Christian Hahnemann (1755-1843). It was based on his formula, "similibus cyrentur," like cures like. Homeopathy is of even greater significance to our time, because it works through the immune system, using nontoxic doses of substances which are similar to those causing the illness. Even today,

Queen Elizabeth is still treated by her personal homeopathic physician at Buckingham Palace. Yet, in the United States, organized medicine continues its frenetic drive to discredit and stamp out the practice of homeopathic medicine. Ironically, Dr. George H. Simmons, who dominated the American Medical Association from 1899 to 1924, building that organization into a national power, had for years run advertisements in Lincoln, Nebraska, where he practiced, which proclaimed that he was a "homeopathic physician."

Clinical trials have shown that homeopathy is as effective as certain widely prescribed arthritic drugs, and also having the overriding advantage that it produces no harmful side effects.

However, the accomplishments of homeopathy have historically been given the silent treatment, or, if mentioned at all, were greatly misinterpreted or distorted. A classic case of this technique occurred in England during the devastating outbreak of cholera in 1854; records showed that during this epidemic, deaths at homeopathic hospitals were only 16.4%, as compared to the death rate of 50% at the orthodox medical hospitals. This record was deliberately suppressed by the Board of Health of the City of London.

During the nineteenth century, the practice of homeopathy spread rapidly throughout the United States and Europe. Dr. Hahnemann had written a textbook, "Homeopathica Materia Medica," which enabled many practitioners to adopt his methods.

In 1847, when the American Medical Association was founded in the United States, homeopaths outnumbered allopaths, the AMA type of doctors, by more than two to one. Because of the individualistic nature of the homeopathic profession, and the fact that they usually practiced alone, they were unprepared for the concerted onslaught of the allopaths. From its beginning, the AMA proved that it was merely a trade lobby, which had been organized for the purpose of stifling competition and driving the homeopaths out of business. By the early 1900s, as the AMA began to achieve this goal, American medicine began to enter its Dark Age. Only now is it beginning to emerge from those decades of darkness, as a new, holistic movement calls for treating the entire physical system, instead of concentrating on one affected part.

A distinctive feature of the AMA's allopathic school of medicine was its constant self-advertisement and promotion of a myth, the myth that its type of medicine was the only one which was effective. This pernicious development created a new monster, the mad doctor as a person of absolute infallibility, whose judgment must never be questioned. Most certainly, his mistakes must never be mentioned. As Ivan Ilyich has pointed out in his shocking book, "Medical Nemesis, the Expropriation of Health" (1976), not only has the effectiveness of the allopathic school of medicine proved to be the stuff of mythology, but the doctors have now brought new plagues into being, illnesses which Ilyich defines as "iatrogenic," causing a plague which he terms "iatrogenesis." Ilyich claims that this plague is now sweeping this nation. He defines iatrogenesis as an "illness which is caused by a doctor's medical intervention." Ilyich goes on to define three commonly encountered types of iatrogenesis; clinical iatrogenesis, which is a doctor-made illness; social iatrogenesis, which is deliberately created by the machinations of the medical-industrial complex; and cultural iatrogenesis, which saps the peoples will to survive. Of the three types of iatrogenesis, the third may be the most prevalent. Advertisements for various medications call it "stress," the difficulty of surmounting the problems of every day life which are caused by the totalitarian government and the sinister figures behind it, who operate it for their own personal gain.

15

Confronted with this monstrous presence, which intrudes into every aspect of an American citizen's daily life, many people are overcome by a feeling of hopelessness, and are persuaded that there is nothing they can do. In fact, this monster is extremely vulnerable, because it is so greatly overextended, and when attacked, can be seen to be a paper tiger.

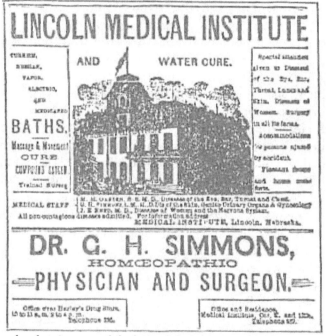

Quack advertisement of the boss of the american medical association

This advertisement appeared in the Lincoln, Nebraska, newspapers years before be obtained his mail order diploma from Rush Medical College. In this license "Doc" Simmons represents himself as a homeopath. He grew more ambitious in his later advertisements and claimed to be a "licentiate of Gynecology and Obstetrics from the Rotuuda Hospitals,

Dublin. Ireland". Note the humbug "Compound Oxygen" Cure.

Despite the AMA's frenetic claims of improving medical care, records show that the state of American health is declining. During the nineteenth century, it had shown steady improvement, probably because of the ministrations of the homeopaths. A typical disease of the period was tuberculosis. In 1812, the death rate from tuberculosis in New York was 700 per 100,000. When Koch isolated the bacillus in 1882, this death rate had already declined to 370. In 1910, when the first TB sanatarium was opened, this rate had further declined to 180 per 100,000. By 1950, this death rate had dropped to 50 per 100,000. Medical records prove that a 90% decline in child mortality from scarlet fever, diptheria, whooping cough and measles occurred before the introduction of antibiotics and immunization, from 1860-1896. This was also well before the Food and Drug Act was passed in 1905, which set up governmental control of interstate commerce in drugs. In 1900, there was only one doctor for every 750 Americans. They had usually served a two year apprenticeship, after which they could look forward to earning about the same salary as a good mechanic. In 1900, the *AMA Journal,* which was already under the editorship of Dr. George H. Simmons, sounded the call to arms. "The growth of the profession must be stemmed if individual members are to find the practice of medicine a lucrative profession." One would find difficulty in reading in the literature of any profession a more determined demand for monopoly. But how was this goal to be achieved? The Merlin who was to wave his magic wand and bring about this dramatic development in the medical profession turned out to be none other than the richest man in the world, the insatiable monopolist, John D. Rockefeller. Fresh from his triumph of organizing his gigantic oil monopoly, a victory as well-blooded as any ancient Roman triumph, Rockefeller, the creature of the House of

Rothschild and its Wall Street emissary, Jacob Schiff, realized that a medical monopoly might bring him even greater profits than his oil trust. In 1892, Rockefeller appointed Frederick T. Gates as his agent, conferring upon him the title of "head of all his philanthropic endeavors." As it turned out, each of Rockefeller's well-publicized "philanthropies" was specifically designed to increase not only his wealth and power, but also the wealth and power of the hidden figures whom he so ably represented.

Frederick T. Gates' first present to Rockefeller was a plan to dominate the entire medical education system in the United States. The initial step was taken by the organization of the Rockefeller Institute of Medical Research. In 1907, the AMA "requested" the Carnegie Foundation to conduct a survey of all the medical schools of the nation. Even at this early date, the Rockefeller interests had already achieved substantial working control of the Carnegie Foundations which has been maintained ever since. It is well known in the foundation world that the Carnegie Foundations (there are several), are merely feeble adjuncts of the Rockefeller Foundation. The Carnegie Foundation named one Abraham Flexner to head up its study of medical schools. Coincidentally, his brother Simon was the head of the Rockefeller Institute of Medical Research. The Flexner Report was completed in 1910, after many months of travel and study. It was heavily influenced by the German-trained allopathic representation in the American medical profession. It was later revealed that the primary influence on Flexner had been his trip to Baltimore. He had been a graduate of Johns Hopkins University. This school had been established by Daniel Coit Gilman (1831- 1908). Gilman had been one of the three original incorporators of the Russell Trust at Yale University (now known as the Brotherhood of Death). Its Yale headquarters had a letter in German authorizing Gilman to set up this branch of the Illuminati in the United States. Gilman incorporated the Peabody Fund and the John Slater Fund, which later became the Rockefeller Foundation. Gilman also became an original incorporator of Rockefeller's General Education Board, which was to take over the United States system of medical education; the Carnegie Foundation and the Russell Sage Foundation. At Johns Hopkins University. Gilman also taught Richard Ely, who became the evil genius of Woodrow Wilson's education. Gil man's final achievement in the last year of his life was to advise Herbert Hoover on the advisability of setting up a think tank. Hoover later followed Gilman's plan in setting up the Hoover Institution after the First World War. This institution furnished the movers and shapers of the "Reagan Revolution" in Washington. Not surprisingly, the American people found themselves saddled with even more debt and an even more oppressive federal bureaucracy, all the result of Daniel Coit Gilman's Illuminati prospectus.

Flexner spent much of his time at Johns Hopkins University finalizing his report. The medical school, which had only been established in 1893, was considered to be very up-to-date. It was also the headquarters of the German allopathic school of medicine in the United States. Flexner, born in Louisville, Ky., had studied at the University of Berlin. The president of the Zionist Organization of America, Louis Brandies, also from Louisville, was an old friend of the Flexner family. After Woodrow Wilson appointed Brandeis to the Supreme Court, Brandeis appointed himself a delegate to Paris to attend the Versailles Peace Conference in 1918. His purpose was to advance the goals of the Zionist movement at this conference.

Bernard Flexner, who was then an attorney in New York, was asked to accompany Brandeis as the official legal counsel to the Zionist delegation in Paris. Bernard Flexner later became a founding member of the Council on Foreign

Relations, and a trustee of the Rockefeller Foundation with his brother Simon.

Simon Flexner had been appointed the first director of the Rockefeller Institute of Medical Research at its organization in 1903. Abraham Flexner joined the Carnegie Foundation for the Advancement of Teaching in 1908, serving there until his retirement in 1928. He also served for years as a member of Rockefeller's General Education Board. He was awarded a Rhodes Memorial lectureship at Oxford University. His definitive work was published in 1913, "Prostitution in Europe."

Abraham Flexner submitted a final report to Rockefeller which apparently was satisfactory in every way. Its first point was an emphatic agreement with the AMA's lament that there were too many doctors. The Flexner solution was a simple one; to make medical education so elitist and expensive, and so drawn out, that most students would be prohibited from even considering a medical career. The Flexner program set up requirements for four years of undergraduate college, and a further four years of medical school. His report also set up complex requirements for the medical schools; they must have expensive laboratories and other equipment. As the requirements of the Flexner Report became effective, the number of medical schools was rapidly reduced. By the end of World War I, the number of medical schools had been reduced from 650 to a mere 50 in number. The number of annual graduates had been reduced from 7500 to 2500. The enactment of the Flexner restrictions virtually guaranteed that the Medical Monopoly in the United States would result in a small group of elitist students from well to do families, and that this small group would be subjected to intense controls.

What has the Flexner Report cost the average American citizen? Some recent statistics throw light on the situation.

The New York Times reported that in 1985, the cost of health care per person in the United States was $1800 per year; in England, $800 per year; in Japan, $600 per year. Yet both England and Japan rank higher on the scale of quality of medical care than the United States.

Compared to Japan, for instance, which has a higher living standard than the United States, but which furnished its citizens with quality medical care for $600 per person each year, comparative medical care in the United States cannot be valued higher than $500 per year per person. What is the $1300 per person difference? It is the $300 billion per year looting of the American public by the Medical Monopoly, in overcharges, criminal syndicalist activities, and the operations of the Drug Trust.

Chapter 2

Quacks on Quackery

Quack—an ignorant pretender to medical or surgical skill.

Quackery—charlatanry. 1783, Crabbe, Village 1, "A potent quack, long versed in human ills, who first insults the victim whom he kills."

Oxford English Dictionary

The first significant figure in American medicine, according to Geoffrey Marks, was the theologian Cotton Mather (1663-1728).

The son of Increase Mather, the President of Harvard University, Cotton Mather wrote many theological works, but also wrote a full length medical work, "The Angel of Bethesda" on which he wrote from 1720 to 1724. His medical letters drew heavily on local Indian lore; he also pondered the mental factor in illness, noting that "A cheerful Heart does Good like a Medicine, but a broken Spirit dries the Bones."

Mather seems to have been the first and last theologian to be interested in the practice of American medicine. The next figure of importance in American medicine was a Dr. Nathan Smith Davis (1817-1904). After apprenticing under Dr. Daniel Clark in upstate New York, Davis moved to New York in 1847. As early as 1845, he had demanded that the Medical Society of the State of New York correct the more flagrant abuses in medical education, insisting that the four months of instruction then in vogue be increased to a period of six months. On May 11, 1846, he convened a group of physicians in New York to form the nucleus of the American Medical Association. The organization took on formal status the following year in Philadelphia, on May 5, 1847, the official date the American Medical Association came into being. The hundred delegates to the New York meeting had swelled to over two hundred and fifty at Philadelphia. They soon formed state organizations in a number of states. Smith later moved to Chicago, where he joined the faculty of Rush Medical School. In 1883, when the AMA founded its Journal, he became the first editor, serving until 1889.

Despite the good intentions of its founder, Dr. Davis, the AMA remained moribund for some fifty years. In 1899, the organization took a giant step forward, with the arrival of one Dr. George H. Simmons from Nebraska. Simmons, who throughout his life was known, perhaps derisively, as "Doc," is now remembered as the pre- eminent American quack. Born in Moreton, England, Simmons immigrated to the United States in 1870. Settling in the Midwest, he began his career as a journalist. It is interesting that the two other dominant figures in twentieth century American medicine, Dr. Morris Fishbein and Albert Lasker, also began their careers as journalists; Fishbein remained a journalist all his life. Simmons became the editor of the *Nebraska Farmer* in Lincoln, Nebraska. Several years later, he decided to improve his finances by launching on a career of unparalleled medical quackery. Interestingly enough, the AMA in 1868 had formally defined quackery as "the sale or administration of drugs or treatments that are not approved by legally constituted medical authorities." Simmons ignored this requirement. No one has ever been able to determine that he had studied anywhere to qualify for a medical degree. Nevertheless, he began to advertise that he was a "licentiate of the Rotunda Hospital of Dublin," referring, presumably, to Dublin, Ireland. In fact, Dublin Hospital had never issued any licenses, nor was it authorized to do so. (See Illustration No. 2, full page opposite.)

No one ever bothered to raise the question as to why Simmons, who had supposedly arrived in the United States as a duly licensed physician, chose instead to practice journalism for some years. He also advertised that he had spent "a year and a half in the largest hospitals in London," although he refrained from making any claims as to what capacity whether as a patient, an orderly or other functionary. Years later, he obtained a diploma by mail from one of the nation's flourishing diploma mills, Rush Medical College in Chicago, while maintaining a full time medical practice in Lincoln. There is no record that he ever set foot on the campus of Rush Medical College prior to obtaining this degree. His protege, Morris Fishbein, also attended Rush Medical College. There was some question as to whether Fishbein ever actually graduated; years later, in his time of influence, he became a "professor" there, specializing in teaching the public relations aspects of medicine.

In their definitive work, "The Story of Medicine in America," an exhaustive and detailed compilation, the authors, Geoffrey Marks and William K. Beatty, make no mention of either Simmons or Fishbein, seemingly a glaring omission, as they are the two most notorious practitioners in our medical history. Apparently realizing that these two men were the two most famous quacks in medical history, the authors prudently decided to ignore them.

In *Who's Who* Simmons notes that he practiced medicine in Lincoln from 1884 to 1899. He lists his degree as L. M. Dublin 1884. This raises further questions. Simmons had immigrated to the United States in 1870; he remained continuously in Lincoln from 1870 to 1899, when he went to Chicago. For some reason, he forebore the listing of the mail order diploma from Rush Medical College in his *Who's Who* listing in the 1936 edition; he had listed it in the 1922 edition as receiving it in 1892. Here again, no one later raised the question of his educational record, which showed that he only began his medical education in Dublin after he had come to the United States. "Doc" Simmons' advertisements in Lincoln, which we have reproduced here, employed a standard phraseology of the time, "A limited number of lady patients can be accommodated at my residence." This was a coded notification that he was engaged in the practice of abortion. He also operated a beauty and massage parlor on the premises, as part of a "Lincoln Institute" of which he was apparently the only official. His advertisements also identified him as a "homeopathic physician," although he would soon embark on a career with the AMA to destroy the profession of homeopathy in the United States. His advertisements announced that he "treats all medical and surgical diseases of women."

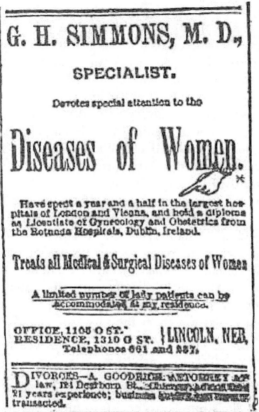

Quack advertisement of the organizer and boss of the american medical association in format used by abortionists The lines, "A limited number of lady patients can be accommodated at my residence," was the form regularly used by abortionists in their advertising in those days. The London and Vienna hospital experienced the Irish license are fictitious. This advertisement appeared at a later date than that Lincoln Institute, but years before "Doc" Simmons had obtained his diploma mill degree.

Having learned about the American Medical Association, Simmons, always in search of more status, formed a Nebraska chapter, the Nebraska Medical Association. His talents as an organizer came to the attention of the Chicago headquarters, and he was summoned to take over the editorship of the Journal of the AMA. Thus "Doc" Simmons came to the AMA, not as a physician, but as a journalist. He found that the AMA was drifting along, with no one capable of implementing a national policy. The situation was made to order for a man of his capacities and drive. He soon named himself as secretary and general manager of the American Medical Association, launching the organization on its dictatorial and self- aggrandizing policies which it has maintained to the present day. All moneys accruing to the AMA passed through Simmons' hands, and he personally supervised every detail of the operations. He soon found an able and willing lieutenant in a man who had formerly served as a Secretary of the Kentucky State Board of Health. He seems to have been a man after Simmons' own heart, for he had been arrested after examiners found a shortage of some $62,000 in his accounts. As a member in good standing of the state bureaucracy, he managed to obtain an official pardon from the Governor of Kentucky, with the gentle admonition that it might be best for him to settle elsewhere. Chicago was only a short train ride away, where he found that Simmons was overwhelmed by his credentials. This gentleman, Dr. E. E. Hyde, died in 1912 from leukemia. This proved to be a fortuitious circumstance for another journalist waiting in the wings, Dr. Morris Fishbein. Fishbein had apparently completed his studies at Rush Medical College, but he had not yet been awarded his diploma. In any case, he did not want to become a doctor. He had desultorily served as an intern at Durand Hospital for a few months, but he was unwilling to comply with the then regulations requiring a two year internship in an accredited hospital. He was seriously considering a career as a circus acrobat, and had been working part time as an extra in an opera company. He had also learned of a possible opening at the AMA, and had been doing some part time writing there during Dr. Hyde's terminal illness. Simmons had also found Fishbein to be a man after his own heart.

When Dr. Hyde died. Simmons at once offered the youth a very handsome starting salary of $100 a month, a high figure for 1913. Fishbein found a home at the AMA; he did not leave until 1949, when he was literally kicked out.

With the advent of Fishbein, the American Medical Association was now firmly in the hands of the nation's two most aggressive quacks, Simmons, who had practised medicine for years, unembarrassed by the fact that he had no medical degree which would hold up under the light of day, and Morris Fishbein, who admitted under oath in 1938 that he had never practised medicine a day in his life. Because "Doc" Simmons, as he was genially known, had never shown any motivation in his career except greed, he soon realized that the enormous power of which the AMA was capable had in effect launched him into a gold mine. He was not slow to request certain considerations in return for the favor or the goodwill of the AMA. First and foremost was its "Seal of Approval" for new products. Since the AMA early on had virtually no laboratory, testing equipment or research staff, the Seal of Approval was obtained by "green research," that is, the laborious determination of how much the supplicant could afford to pay, and how much it might be worth to him. At first, some pharmaceutical manufacturers resented this arrangement, and refused to pay. The leader of this opposition was one Dr. Wallace C. Abbott, who had founded Abbott Laboratories in 1900. Simmons met him head on by refusing to approve a single product of Abbott Laboratories, no matter how many were submitted. This standoff continued for some time, until one morning, "Doc" Simmons was visibly shaken to see Dr. Abbott towering over him in his office.

"Well, sir," he stammered, "and just what can I do for you?" "I just came down to hear from you personally" Dr. Abbott replied, "why not one of my products has ever been approved by the AMA."

"That's not really my department, sir," "Doc" Simmons replied, "I'll be glad to check with our research department and find out what the problem is."

"Is there any way I could speed up your inquiry?" asked Dr. Abbott.

Simmons was overjoyed. At last the stubborn chemist was beginning to see things his way. "I'll be glad to do whatever I can," he said. "There is something you can do," said Dr. Abbott, "if you would be so good as to look over these documents, it might help you to make up your mind."

He spread a number of papers out on "Doc" Simmons' desk. Simmons immediately realized that he was looking at a complete record of his career, carefully garnered by private detectives who had been hired by Dr. Abbott. There were the full details of the so- called "diplomas'; records of sex charges brought against Simmons by former patients in Lincoln, and other titillating items, such as charges of medical negligence resulting in the deaths of patients. He knew that he was trapped.

"All right," said Simmons, "just what is it you want?"

"All I want is to have the AMA grant approval of my products," said Dr. Abbott. "Do you think that is possible, now?"

"You've got it," said Simmons. From that day, the products from Abbott's firm, which was still called Abbott Biologicals at that time, were rushed through the AMA process and marked "Approved." Dr. Abbott never paid one cent for this special treatment.

Through the years, various versions of the Abbott-Simmons conflict were repeated. A whitewashed version appears in Tom Mahoney's "Merchants of Life," which claims that Simmons objected to Dr. Abbott's "commercialization" of the medical profession, and wished to teach him a lesson. The Council on Pharmacy and Chemistry not only refused to approve any of Abbott's drugs, but also turned down his requests to advertise in the journal of the American Medical Association, and later refused to print his letters of protest. Simmons then launched personal attacks on Dr. Abbott in the Journal in the issues of December 1907 and March 1908. Simmons' pious claim that he did not wish to see Dr. Abbott commercializing the medical profession rings hollow; Abbott was manufacturing pharmaceutical products for sale. The rub was that he refused to pay the usual shakedown to Simmons.

After the imbroglio was settled, S. DeWitt Clough, Abbott's advertising manager, became a bridge playing crony of Morris Fishbein.

A spirited critic of the AMA during its Simmons-Fishbein period, Dr. Emanuel Josephson of New York, wrote, "The methods which Simmons and his crew used in their battle for a monopoly of medical publications and of advertisements to the profession were often crude and illegitimate. The AMA has openly threatened firms that advertise in media other than their own journals with withdrawal of 'acceptance' of their products." Dr. Josephson described Simmons' practices as "conspiracy in restraint of trade, and extortion." He further charged, again correctly, that "almost every branch of the Federal Government active in the field of medicine was completely dominated by the Association." This was borne out by the present writer, who cites many instances later of government agencies actively implementing the most horrendous cases of racketeering by the Drug Trust. So exhaustive were the controls set in place by Simmons that the President of the AMA, Dr. Nathan B.

van Etten, later filed a sworn affidavit in the New York District Court that he, as President of the American Medical Association, had no authority to accept any moneys or enter into any contracts. All such deals were the province of the Chicago headquarters staff. It was later noted that AMA "focuses on protecting physicians' incomes against government intrusion in the practice of medicine." This was a case of having their cake and eating it too. While steadfastly opposing any government supervision of the Medical Monopoly, the monopolists frequently forced various government agencies to act against anyone who posed a threat to their monopoly, having them arrested, prosecuted, and sent to prison.

"Doc" Simmons' lucrative dominance of the American Medical Association led him into numerous sidelines. In 1921, he established the Institute of Medicine in Chicago. This apparently was nothing more than a holding company for his bribes. He had also been enjoying the perquisites of the American success story, a buxom mistress installed in a luxurious Gold Coast apartment. Scoundrel that he was, Simmons was not content to flaunt this liason to his wife; he also became increasingly cruel in his determination to get rid of her. He then embarked on a classic ploy, the physician attempting to dispose of an unwanted wife by plying her with narcotics, trying to convince her that she is going insane, and hopefully, driving her to suicide. After some months of this treatment, his wife fought back by filing suit against him. A highly publicized trial in 1924 ended in his wife's testimony that he had given her heavy doses of narcotics, prescribed on the strength of his "medical experience," and then began proceedings to have her declared insane. This was not such an unusual procedure during that period; it had happened to literally hundreds of wives. However, his wife proved to be tougher than most victims. She testified in court that he had tried to have her framed on a charge of insanity. This trial inspired more than a dozen subsequent books, plays, and movies based on the story of a physician who tries to drive his wife insane through a campaign of ministration of drugs and psychological terrorism. The most famous was "Gaslight," in which Charles Boyer played the role of "Doc" Simmons to perfection, the luckless wife being played by Ingrid Bergman.

The trial brought Simmons a torrent of unpleasant publicity, and forced his retirement as head of the AMA. However, he retained the title of "general editor emeritus," absenting himself in 1924 until his death in 1937. Morris Fishbein, still operating under his lucky star, was now moved into total dominance of the AMA. Between the two of them, they controlled the AMA for more than a half century, perfecting their techniques for using this organization to raise money, exercise political clout, and maintain dominance over physicians, hospitals, drug companies and concerned government agencies. Simmons moved to Hollywood, Florida, where he lived until 1937. His *New York Times* obituary was headlined "Noted for War on Quacks." His longtime critic, Dr. Emanuel Josephson, noted that this was an odd memorial for a man who had long been known as "the Prince of Quacks."

Morris Fishbein also inherited Simmons' able assistant at the AMA, Dr. Olin West (1874-1952). West had been state director in Tennessee for the Rockefeller Sanitary Commission from 1910 to 1918. Thus he had the requisite credentials as a representative of the Rockefeller connection at the AMA headquarters. Dr. Josephson later termed Fishbein "the Hitler of the medical profession" and West as "his Goering." Fishbein remained aware of the AMA's ability to "use" government employees for AMA purposes. Of the first fifteen members of the Council on Pharmacy and Chemistry, three had been members of the federal government.

With the disappearance of Simmons, Fishbein now had a free hand. From that day on, he made sure that when anyone mentioned the AMA, they also paid tribute to Morris Fishbein. He used his position there to launch a host of private enterprises, including book publishing, lecturing, and writing feature newspaper columns. On a very modest salary of $24,000 a year from the AMA, Fishbein became the Playboy of the Western World. His children were supervised by a French governess, while he commuted weekly to New York to be seen at the Stork Club and to attend first nights at the theatre. Fees, kickbacks, awards and other moneys poured into his coffers in a veritable flood. During his twenty-five years of power at the AMA, he never lost an opportunity to advertise and enrich himself. Despite the fact that he had never practiced medicine a day in his life, he persuaded King Features Syndicate to sign him on as daily columnist writing a "medical" commentary which appeared in over two hundred newspapers. A full page ad appeared in *Editor and Publisher* to celebrate his new venture on March 23, 1940, stating "An authority of medicine, Dr. Fishbein's name is synonymous with the 'sterling' stamp on a piece of silver." Whether this was an oblique reference to Judas is not clear.

Fishbein garnered additional income by having himself named medical adviser to *Look* Magazine, the second largest publication in the United States. In 1935, he had ventured into what was probably his greatest financial coup, the annual publication of a massive volume, "the Modern Home Medical Adviser." The book was written for him by doctors on consignment, but he wrote the lurid advertising copy, "Endorsed by doctors everywhere. The Wealthiest Millionaire Could Not Buy Better Health Guidance." Obviously, no doctor anywhere dared to criticize the book.

Fishbein's steadily aggrandizing powers at the AMA were veiled by the fact that he never had any title there except "editor." He maintained absolute control over all the publications of the AMA, and thus gained his total power over the organization. No one who disagreed with him had any opportunity to voice any discontent. He also maintained absolute control over the selection of the personnel of the various committees of the AMA, so that no one was ever in a position to attack him. The Committee on Food and the Council on Pharmacy and Chemistry were his particular preserves, because of the great power they had over manufacturers and advertisers. The Council on Pharmacy and Chemistry had been set up in 1905, at the same time that the Food and Drug Act had been passed by congress; the two groups always worked together very closely. As advertising revenues increased each year, Fishbein steadfastly denied that any profits were being made by the AMA. He was quoted in *Review of Reviews,* 1926, "Far from being the 'corporation not for profit' which the statutes list it, the American Medical Association has been exceedingly profitable to the public, both in dollars and in lives." Thus Fishbein adeptly turned aside growing criticism of the income of the AMA by his claim that it was profitable to the public at large.

Under Fishbein's editorship, the AMA health magazine, *Hygiea,* carried the banner headline, "PURE FOODS, HONESTLY ADVERTISED." "The Seal of Acceptance of the Committee on Foods of the AMA is your best guarantee that the claims of quality for any product are correct and that the advertising for it is truthful. Look for this Seal on every food that you buy. White Star Tuna and Chicken of the Sea brand Tuna have this acceptance." At the very time that Fishbein was running these advertisements, the Food and Drug Administration was repeatedly seizing shipments of these very brands of tuna, condemning them because "they consisted in whole or in part of decomposed animal substance." So much for the Seal of Acceptance.

The AMA Committee on Foods always verged on the brink of exposure or serious damage suits, because it had virtually no testing apparatus. The June 24, 1931 issue of *Business Week* raised serious questions about these operations, particularly the power of the AMA to censor manufacturers' ad copy. *Business Week* asked "whether a national body of professional men conducted presumably on the highest ethical plane, is not continually exceeding the natural boundaries of its actions when it attempts to assume police and regulatory powers over the nation's largest industry." The editors of *Business Week* were well aware that the staff at AMA did little testing and were not qualified to render judgments on the "acceptance" of products. The magazine story may have been intended as a quiet warning to the AMA to cease and desist its activities in this field. They reckoned without Fishbein's chutzpah. The AMA Committee on Foods, under Fishbein's guidance, continued its operations for another decade. In 1939, Fishbein awarded the Seal of Acceptance to some 2,706 individual products, which were produced by some 1,653 companies. Its chief rival in this field, the Good Housekeeping Seal of Approval, had also come under increasing fire for its aggressive tactics in seeking more customers for its Seal. In May 1941, the Federal Trade Commission issued "cease and desist" orders against the Good Housekeeping Seal; Fishbein saw the handwriting on the wall, and shortly afterwards, he discontinued the AMA Seal of Acceptance awards for general purpose foods.

The Council on Pharmacy and Chemistry was quite another matter. This was the key to the big money. A drug company could make one hundred million dollars on a new product, if it were to be released under the proper auspices; the most vital, of course, was the AMA Seal of Acceptance. The opportunities for large scale bribery, conspiracy and corruption were too prevalent to be ignored. One physician who was very conscious of this was Dr. Emanuel Josephson of New York. Heir to a large fortune, Dr. Josephson resided in a multi-million dollar townhouse in the city's most expensive area, just around the corner from Nelson Rockefeller on the fashionable Upper East Side. Josephson was unable to conceal his contempt for Fishbein and his money-grubbing activities. On January 2, 1932, he officially resigned from the AMA's New York City Medical Society; the AMA chose to ignore his letter of resignation until 1938, when Fishbein released a letter claiming that the AMA "had severed connections with him." In 1939, Dr. Josephson submitted the important record of his ground breaking research to *Science Magazine*, "Vitamin E Therapy of Myasthenia Gravis," which they refused to print. Dr. Josephson later pointed out that the AMA had deliberately concealed the benefits of Vitamin E therapy for more than twenty-five years. This was only one instance of hundreds in which the AMA withheld life-saving information from the public. The benefits of Vitamin E therapy are now generally recognized by the medical profession.

The AMA technique for controlling all new products was revealed by a United Press dispatch January 20, 1940, that the AMA had a well-defined newspaper policy "never to call anything a cure, or in fact give publicity to any remedy of any description, without a thorough investigation." The organization usually recommended that any report of a remedy should be referred to the New York branch of the AMA for investigation. As Dr. Josephson testified, he had tried for years to get the New York chapter of the AMA to investigate his findings, but they always refused.

The AMA Council on Pharmacy and Chemistry had effectively solidified its control by amending the official AMA Code of Ethics to prohibit individual physicians from giving any testimonials in favor of any drug; this amendment protected the valuable monopoly of AMA headquarters in Chicago. A distinguished scientist and teacher, Dr. Frank G.

Lydston, published a booklet, "Why the AMA is Going Backward," in which he stated, "The achievement of what the oligarchy of the AMA has boasted most vociferously has been its belated war on proprietaries, quack medical manufacturers and unproved products. When I recall the nauseous array of proprietary fakes on the advertisements on which the oligarchy built its financial prosperity, its 'holier than thou' pose is sickening. It was fitting to its psychic constitution that after the AMA has for years done its level best to promulgate the interests, and to fatten upon, fake manufacturers and professional poisoners of the innocent, it should bite the hand that fed it. Despotic powers such as the oligarchy wields over the food and drug manufacturers is dangerous, and human nature being what it is, that power might be expected to sooner or later to be abused."

Dr. Josephson also observed that "The history of the AMA's Seal of Acceptance is replete with betrayals of professional and public trust. Drug products of the highest value have been rejected or their acceptance unwarrantedly delayed. Worthless, dangerous or deadly food and drugs have been hastily accepted."

On April 20, 1936, *Time* magazine reported that the American Medical Association was then worth $3,800,000, of which two million was in government bonds, one million in cash, with an $800,000 headquarters building in Chicago. *Time* also mentioned another little known aspect of the AMA medical monopoly, "Shoes designed to correct foot trouble must be approved by AMA before a conscientious physician may prescribe them." Just how the AMA had set up this shoe monopoly was not clear.

On July 7, 1961, *Time* reported that the AMA *Journal* now had a circulation of 180,000, with income of 16 million dollars a year, "the bulk from ads in its publications mainly by drug and appliance makers." The AMA Constitution states that it was organized "to promote the art and science of medicine and the betterment of public health." Yet the history of the AMA was replete with events which contradicted this goal. *Literary Digest* reported on June 11, 1927, the AMA had adopted a resolution that alcohol had no scientific place in medicine. In all fairness, it should be reported that the 1917 resolution had probably been passed at the behest of the Rockefeller interests, which, for their own hidden purposes, were strongly supporting passage of prohibition at that time.

On February 9, 1977, the Federal Trade Commission issued an order against the AMA because it had barred certain drug advertisements. Throughout the 25-year reign of Morris Fishbein at the AMA, the organization repeatedly made bewildering about face recommendations on certain products, the reason for such reversals being known only by Fishbein himself. The situation also offered impressive profits to be made by investing in the stock of a certain drug firm just before it received the coveted AMA Seal of Acceptance for a new product. After such an announcement, it was not unusual for the stock of the drug firm to double in price. Only Dr. Fishbein knew when such an approval would be released.

One of the more reprehensible decisions made by Dr. Fishbein during his long reign at the AMA was his move to hush up a dangerous outbreak of amoebic dysentery in Chicago at the height of the World's Fair observance in 1933. Although the cause of the outbreak was traced to faulty plumbing at the Congress Hotel, Fishbein met with a group of Chicago business leaders and pledged the cooperation of the AMA in holding back any warnings until the Fair had ended its season. Hundreds of unsuspecting tourists who visited the World's Fair returned to their home towns infected with the terrible illness, which often lingers for years, and is very difficult to treat or to cure.

The list of dangerous drugs approved by Fishbein during his tenure as public spokesman for the AMA is lengthy and terrifying. Fishbein hastened to approve the notorious diet drug, dinetrophenol, despite laboratory records that it was dangerous to health. Another drug, tryparsamide, manufactured by Merck under license from the Rockefeller Institute for Medical Research, was a dangerous arsenical drug. Used to counter the effects of syphilis, it was abandoned by its discoverer, Paul Ehrlich, when he found that it caused blindness by atrophying the optic nerve. Ehrlich's warnings did not prevent the AMA, Merck or the Rockefeller Institute from continuing to distribute this drug.

In the issue of June 21, 1937, Morris Fishbein had a cover portrait on *Time* magazine. It was an unusually unflattering photograph, in which Fishbein looked as though he needed a doctor. *Time* had published a story earlier that year that Fishbein was suffering from Bell's Palsy. The right side of his face hung slack, and he was obviously in very poor condition.

One of Fishbein's most dangerous errors was his approval of sulfathiazole in 1941. On January 25, 1941, Fishbein announced that Winthrop Drug Company's sulfathiazole "has been accepted by the Council on Pharmacy and Chemistry for inclusion in its official volume of new and non-official remedies." Winthrop was a subsidiary of the international drug cartel, I. G. Farben.

Sulfathiazole was also approved by Dr. J. J. Durrett, the FDA official in charge of new drugs. Durrett was a Rockefeller-approved appointee to this vital position. By December 1940, 400,000 tablets had been sold, which contained as much as 5 grains each of Luminal. The safe dosage was 1 grain of Luminal. Many persons who took the Winthrop dosage never woke up.

In 1937, the AMA approved an extremely poisonous preparation of sulfanilamide in a solution of diethylene glucol; this mixture caused a number of fatalities. It caused white blood cell loss, even though it was advertised that it would "help" heart disease. Long after Fishbein's departure, the AMA continued to endorse potentially dangerous products. The Winter issue of the *Journal* of the American Medical Association featured advertisements for Suprol in 200 mg capsules (suprofen), an analgesic which had been approved by the FDA in December of 1985. It was produced by McNeil, a subsidiary of Johnson and Johnson. By February 13, 1986, the firm had received the first reports of acute kidney damage, yet on December 2nd the FDA Arthritis Advisory Board recommended that Suprol remain on sale as an "alternative analgesic." It had already been banned in Denmark, Greece, Ireland, Italy and Great Britain; McNeil suspended its production here on May 15.

One of the more reprehensible episodes in Fishbein's long career was his denial of the Seal of Acceptance of the AMA to sulfanilamide, although it had been saving lives in Europe for several years. Because its producers had failed to negotiate a satisfactory deal with Fishbein, numerous persons in the United States continued to die of septicemia, or blood poisoning. The dam finally broke when a member of the Roosevelt family, in dire need of immediate treatment with sulfanilimide, had his physician obtain a special supply. Shortly thereafter the AMA Council was forced to "accept" it. In 1935 and 1936, the Council accepted and advertised in the *Journal* a heart stimulant, Digitol, at the very time that government agencies were seizing and condemning interstate shipments of this drug as a substance dangerous to life. Another product, Ergot Aseptic, was accepted by the Council, and advertisements for this product prominently featured in the *Journal,* at the same time that government agencies were seizing and condemning its shipments because of adulterants and misbranding.

Under the leadership of the nation's two most notorious quacks, Simmons and Fishbein, a gigantic nationwide drug operation was perfected which today poses a serious threat to the health of every American citizen. The fixed prices of these drugs has been a contributing factor to the meteroric rise in the cost of health care. In 1976, the national bill was 95 billion dollars, which was 8.4% of the Gross National Product, a figure which had risen from 4.5% in 1962. From 1955-1975, the price index rose 74%, while the cost of medical care rose 300%. Dr. Robert S. Mendelsohn, an independent health practitioner, estimates that 30% of Xrays taken in the United States, some 300 million a year, are ordered when there is no valid medical need. A federal expert reports that if we would reduce the unnecessary Xrays by one/third, we could save the lives of one thousand cancer patients each year. Yet the responsible organization, the American Cancer Society, has consistently ignored this problem. The genetic effect of Xrays on the population in a single year has been predicted to cause as many as thirty thousand deaths per year in future years. In 1976, doctors wrote one billion doses for sleeping pills, some twenty-seven million prescriptions which resulted in twenty-five thousand trips to emergency rooms for adverse drug reactions, and some fifteen hundred emergency room deaths from tranquilizers. Ninety per cent of these victims are women. By 1978, five billion tranquilizer pills were being prescribed; the most notorious of these, Valium, produces five hundred million dollars per year income for Hoffman LaRoche Co.; it is the epitome of the mythical "soma" described by Aldous Huxley in his "Brave New World," "the perfect drug, narcotic, pleasantly hallucinant."

An English study showed that aspirin caused fetal defects, deaths, birth defects, and bleeding in newborn babies. Recently, a nationwide campaign was launched proclaiming that new studies "showed" that an aspirin a day would prevent heart attack in men. An appended afterthought suggested that it might be wise to check with a personal physician before embarking on this regimen, but how many thousands of men will at once begin to take a daily aspirin, hoping to postpone a dreaded heart attack, and unaware that they may be suffering from another result of the ingestion of aspirin, internal bleeding? It is this property of thinning the blood which caused it to be recommended as a preventive for heart attack.

Aspirin is also of doubtful value when taken to reduce fever; by reducing fever in some instances, notably during the onset of pneumonia, it disguises the symptoms of pneumonia so that the physician is unable to make this diagnosis. It usually takes twenty minutes to dissolve in the stomach, and then only if it is taken with a full glass, eight ounces, of water. Few people know that if aspirin is taken with orange juice, its efficacy is greatly diminished, because it may not dissolve.

In September of 1980, the Food and Drug Administration announced that it would remove from the market more than three thousand drugs whose effectiveness had not been proven. During the previous year, Americans had spent more than one billion dollars on these same "unproven" drugs, many of which had been "accepted" by the AMA. In 1962, Congress had passed amendments to the Food and Drug Act which implemented drug effectiveness requirements by 1964. The drug manufacturers resisted all attempts to force them to comply with these amendments, forcing the FDA to remove them from the market some sixteen years later. The average life of an effective drug is about fifteen years; this meant that the delaying tactics of the drug manufacturers had allowed them to milk these unproven drugs for their entire effective market life!

We now come to the most amazing record of criminal syndicalism in our history. After Congress had passed stringent requirements in 1962 to force the drug manufacturers to prove that their drugs were effective (a requirement which in many cases was impossible to observe, since they were worthless), the drug manufacturers were advised by their cohorts in the AMA and the advertising industry that it would be wise to start a brushfire, a diversionary tactic which would draw attention from the fact that they had failed to comply with the new Congressional requirements. This diversionary tactic was to be called "the War Against Quackery." A few months after the new regulations went into effect, the AMA Board of Trustees met to create a new committee, the Committee on Quackery, which was formally incorporated on November 2, 1963. It was originally intended to destroy the entire profession of chiropractic in the United States, the nation's second largest health care group. It soon branched out in search of further victims, as the "Coordinating Conference on Health Information." This subsidiary was the brainchild of a New York letterhead outfit called the Pharmaceutical Advertising Council, which in turn was merely a space on the desk of the President of Grey Medical Advertising Company, a wholly owned subsidiary of the prestigious Grey Advertising Company in New York.

Although it was ostensibly merely an advisory group, the Coordinating Conference on Health Information soon launched an all-out war on independent health practitioners all over the United States. Its victims were usually selected by the nonprofit AMA, aided by the charitable foundations, the American Cancer Society and the Arthritis Foundation, both of which had been smarting under accusations that they were killing patients while independent health advisors were saving them. The criminal syndicalists were able to enlist the full police powers of the federal government, through contacts in the Federal Trade Commission, the Post Office Department, the Food and Drug Administration, and the United States Public Health Service. These federal agents were solicited by the charitable foundations to initiate police actions against hundreds of unsuspecting health practitioners throughout the United States. It was one of the most massive, well planned and ruthless operations in which the federal agents ever engaged. In many cases, .people were arrested for selling or sometimes giving away booklets which advised such innocuous health practices as taking vitamins! These distributors now found themselves under restraining orders from the Post Office, the Department of Justice, and the Food and Drug Administration. Others, who were distributing various salves, nostrums and other preparations, most of them based on herbal formulae, received heavy fines and prison sentences. In every case, all of the stocks of these practitioners, many of whom were elderly and impoverished, were seized and destroyed as "dangerous substances." It was never alleged that a single person had ever been injured, much less killed, by any of these preparations. At the same time, the drug manufacturers were continuing to sell drugs which produced extensive side effects such as kidney damage, liver damage and death. Not one of them was ever enjoined from distributing these products on the terms used against the independent health practitioners. In most cases, when these dangerous drugs were banned in the United States, the manufacturers shipped them overseas to countries in Latin America and Asia, where they continue to be sold to this day. The stock of Syntex Corporation rose from a few dollars to a high of $400 a share when it started dumping steroids in foreign markets.

Many of the attacks were focused against the distributors of an anti-cancer preparation called laetrile, a fruit product. Extremely sensitive to any rival of their very profitable chemotherapy drugs, the cancer profiteers ordered the federal agents to carry out terror raids against their competitors. Often striking at night, in groups of heavily armed SWAT teams, the federal agents broke down doors to capture elderly women and their stocks of herbal teas. Many of these housewives and retired persons carried small amounts of vitamins and health preparations which they furnished to neighbors or friends at cost. They had no funds to fight the massed agencies of the federal government, who themselves were merely patsies for the Drug Trust. In many cases, the victims lost their homes, their life savings and all other attachable assets, because they had posed a threat to the Medical Monopoly. It was the most blatant use of the police powers by the Big Rich to protect their profitable enterprises. To this day, most of these victims have no idea that they were knocked off by the Rockefeller Monopoly.

Sidney W. Bishop, deputy postmaster general, boasted at the Second National Congress on Medical Quackery in 1963, "I am particularly proud of the excellent arrangements existing between the Food and Drug Administration, the Federal Trade Commission and the Post Office department to maintain coordination in the exchange of information leading to the establishment of criminal prosecution," a laudatory reference to the success of the "war against quackery." It was later revealed that the Coordinating Conference on Health Information had been entirely financed by the leading drug companies of the Medical Monopoly, Lederle, Hoffman LaRoche and others. From 1964 to 1974, their search and destroy campaign was carried on as a total war by federal agents against anyone who had ever offered any type of health food or health advice. The goal of course, was the elimination of all competition to the major drug companies.

In 1967, the AMA received 43% of its total income, $13.6 million, from its drug advertisements. It then issued a letter of agreement jointly with the Food and Drug Administration publicizing a campaign to "enhance public awareness of health fraud devices and products by identifying them as ineffective and potential health hazards." These were the same persons who had been unable to persuade the drug companies to comply with federal requirements that they prove the effectiveness of their drug products! The hazards, as we have stated, lay more with the Drug Trust than from the elderly ladies in California who were advising people to eat more garlic and lettuce if they wished to stay healthy.

The death tolls were from "approved" drugs, not from the preparations distributed by the holistic health advocates.

The AMA then sponsored a National Health Fraud Conference, whose principle spokesman was Congressman Claude Pepper. This was an ironic turn of events, because a few years earlier, the then Senator Claude Pepper, one of the most powerful political figures in Washington, had aroused the ire of the AMA because he planned to support socialized medicine in the United States. A longtime spokesman for leftwing interests, who was known as "Red" Pepper because of his political sympathies, Pepper had found himself attacked by the big guns and money of the AMA. They found a candidate to oppose him in Nixon's friend, George Smathers, and Pepper was defeated in Florida. Coming back as a Congressman, Pepper now licked the boots of those who had ousted him. He endorsed their police state methods against anyone who dared to challenge the power of the Medical Monopoly.

Having proved his loyalty to the Rockefeller power, Pepper was allowed to stage another health conference in 1984. It was denounced by informed observers as a typical "Moscow show trial." The new Pepper sideshow was called the Congressional Hearings on Quackery. Pepper claimed that "health fraud" was a ten billion dollar a year scandal, an impressive figure for what was essentially a small cottage industry. He summoned a longtime apologist for the Medical Monopoly, Dr. Victor Herbert, a physician at the Bronx Veterans Administration Hospital. Herbert demanded that the Justice Department use the RICO (Racketeer Inspired Criminal Organization) strike force against "medical charlatans" and "health frauds" by using the same techniques which had been employed against organized crime. RICO allows the government to confiscate all assets of those who are convicted "as a result of a proved conspiracy." In December of 1987, this same Dr. Victor Herbert surfaced again, filing a 70 page complaint in the U.S. District Court in Iowa. He charged that the officials of the National Health Federation, a rival to the AMA, and other alternative health care practitioners had libelled him. Kirkpatrick Dilling, the attorney for the defendants, termed the suit a flagrant attempt to destroy freedom of choice in health care in the United States. Dilling pointed out that Herbert was backed by a shadow group called the American Council for Science and Health, a front for major food manufacturing companies.

Dr. Herbert was joined at the Pepper Hearings by a longtime agent of the Medical Monopoly, Mrs. Anna Rosenberg. She voiced her outrage that there should still be any competition in the United States for the Drug Trust. A longtime vassal of the Rockefeller family, she had served as director of the American Cancer Society during its valiant struggle to restrict all treatment to the orthodox and highly profitable "cut, slash and burn" techniques, which, unfortunately for the patients, usually proved to be fatal. Anna Rosenberg had been married to Julius Rosenberg. She earned five thousand dollars a week as "labor relations specialist" to keep unions out of Rockefeller Center and to keep its underpaid minions on the job.

The Coordinating Conference on Health Information ran amuck for some ten years, sending hundreds of victims to prison on what were in most instances flimsy or trumped up charges. The desired effect, to terrorize everyone who had become active in the alternative health care field, was achieved. Most health practitioners went underground, or closed up their businesses; others left the country. An inevitable reaction against these terrorists operations set in; by 1974, there were public demands for a Congressional investigation of the SWAT tactics used by the Post Office and the

U.S. Public Health Service against elderly housewives. Such an investigation would inevitably have revealed that these conscientious and dedicated public servants were actually faceless tools of the sinister behind the scenes figures who manipulated the government of the United States for their own power and profit. Needless to say, no such Congressional investigation was ever held. Instead, the CCHI suddenly went underground. They were immune from countersuits by their victims, because all actions had been taken against the victims by federal agents. They were not immune, according to the statutes, but the chances of recovering against them in any federal court was remote. (The present writer has on numerous occasions sought redress against federal agents in federal courts, only to have a polite federal judge rule against him in every instance.)

After the Coordinating Conference on Health Information went underground, health practitioners in the State of California suddenly found themselves under more concerted attack than ever before. The activist now was the California State Board of Health. It was then found that the stealthy minions of CCHI, still doing the work of the Medical Monopoly, had merely abandoned their national operations for fear of exposure, but had now nested in the California State Board of Health like a group of diseased rats hiding from inevitable retribution. The CCHI has remained imbedded in the California State Board of Health ever since, carrying on a steady warfare against health practitioners in that state. The drug cartel continued to operate unmolested.

This war against American citizens fulfills every requirement for prosecution under the statutes forbidding criminal syndicalism in the United States. It is a classic case of a supposedly nonprofit organization, the American Medical Association, conspiring with certain charitable foundations, notably the American Cancer Society and the Arthritis Foundation, to enlist public agencies to start a war to benefit the national Drug Trust, while denying American citizens the benefits of reasonably priced and effective health care. Not only were there repeated violations of the constitutional rights of citizens who were active in the health care movement, often from a sense of public service rather than from a desire for profit, while the evidence of an active conspiracy (RICO) to subvert official government agencies for the profit of private multinational drug firms is too abundant to ignore. Those who have been victimized by the CCHI conspiracy can also bring actions against Lederle, Hoffman laRoche and the other drug firms who hired these people to do their dirty work. The trail of liability is plain; it will be simple to establish it in court.

Meanwhile, the effect of the CCHI depredations has been devastating. Millions of Americans, particularly the elderly and the poor, have been forcibly deprived of reasonably priced health care because of this conspiracy. These victims have been forced to do without their modestly priced health advisors, and thrown onto the care of the high-priced physicians from the AMA, who place them on expensive drugs produced by the Rockefeller drug monopoly. The fact that many of these drugs are overpriced, ineffective, and potentially dangerous has been routinely covered up by the federal agencies responsible for protecting the public, particularly the Food and Drug Administration. It is notable that the drug cartels have never been investigated by any government agency under the pertinent provisions of the Sherman Anti-Trust Act, because these cartels are the property of the international financial monopolists.

This proves what many observers have charged for years, that the government regulations purportedly enacted by Congress to protect the public have, in reality, served only to protect the monopolists. By 1986, this Medical Monopoly had reached a yearly take of $355.4 billion a year, eleven per cent of the Gross National Product of the United States. The Medical Monopoly has long had its critics among conscientious members of the medical profession. In December 1922, the *Illinois Medical Journal* featured an article which declared that "The American Medical Association has become an autocracy." This was during the heyday of Dr. Simmons' rule in Chicago. The article denounced the dictatorial assumption of power over the entire medical profession. Although it had first organized in 1847, the AMA had not formally incorporated until 1897, when it paid a three dollar fee to the Secretary of the State of Illinois. Within two years after its incorporation, "Doc" Simmons had arrived on the scene to begin his twenty-five year power grab. He soon realized that the medical schools control the hospitals; the medical examination boards control the medical schools, and so he expanded the power of the AMA until he had total control over the medical examination boards.

The records show that coincidentally with the growing power of the AMA, there came a corresponding decline in the quality of medical care and the personal responsibility of the physicians to their patients. The AMA enacted a stern Code of Ethics, which serve to form a phalanx of protection for any physician who faced criticism for his errors, such errors, in many cases, resulted in the crippling or deaths of his patients. This same "code" usually prevents any physician, nurse or other hospital employee from testifying in court about the errors committed by a physician.

One noted physician, Dr. Norman Barnesby, who had long been a prominent member of the U.S. Army Medical Staff and the U.S. Public Health Service, said, "Chaos and crime is inevitable so long as doctors abide by the AMA's code of ethics, the code of silence. *(This is akin to the notorious Omerta, the code of silence of the Mafia, which invokes the death penalty to any member who reveals the secrets of the Cosa Nostra. The Medical Gnostics, the AMA, has set up its own Cosa Nostra, which passes a sentence of professional death against any physician who reveals any medical omissions or crimes, the result being ostracism from the profession, denial of hospital privileges, and other drastic forms of punishment. Editor's Note.)* The ethics to which doctors subscribe smells to high heavens. It is a disgrace to any vaunting civilization. 'A peculiar reserve must be maintained by physicians toward the public in regard to professional questions and as there exist many points in medical ethics and etiquette through which the feelings of physicians may be painfully assaulted in their intercourse, and which cannot be understood or appreciated by general society, neither the subject matter of their differences nor the adjudication of their arbitration should be made public."

The last part of this paragraph is Dr. Barnesby's direct quote from the AMA Code of Ethics. Note the arrogance of the AMA in claiming that "medical ethics and etiquette" cannot be understood by general society. Dr. Barnesby continues, "I am convinced that the remedy lies in a full abolition of all codes and practices inimical to society, and a complete reorganization of the system on the lines of legal supervision or other responsible control." Dr. Barnesby's recommendations were ignored by the Medical Monopoly.

An AP dispatch of February 11, 1988 noted that "5% of Doctors Lie About Credentials" a headline of facts discovered by a large health care corporation, Humana, Inc., found that 39 of 727 doctors who applied to work in their clinics during a six-month period, that is 5%, presented false credentials. Even worse, many doctors, convicted of drug or sex charges in one state, simply move to another state and set up practice, protected by the Medical Monopoly. There have been horrendous stories in recent years about habitual sex offenders, convicted in one state, who go to another state and through their professional practice, began their career of violating children once more.

A gifted physician, Dr. Ernest Codman, of a distinguished New England family, addressed the annual AMA convention on March 2, 1924 as follows:

"I have notes on four hundred registered cases of supposed bone sarcoma. All of these four hundred registered cases, with few exceptions, are records of error and failure; I have many of the foremost surgeons and pathologists in the country convicted in their own handwriting of gross errors in these cases. Legs have been amputated when they should not have been, and left on when they should have been amputated."

Dr. Codman's speech left his audience dumbfounded. None of them challenged his statements, but his speech was deliberately hushed up by AMA officials. He wryly records that never again during his distinguished professional career was he asked to address any AMA meeting.

From time to time, other dissidents have appeared at AMA meetings, to engage in a brief skirmish as they voiced their objections, and then disappear, forgotten in the all consuming war to maintain the Medical Monopoly. *Time* magazine gave a brief summary of one such episode on June

6, 1970, with the headline, "Schizophrenic AMA." The story noted that some thirty to forty dissidents, young idealistic doctors, had rushed the podium and taken over the AMA annual meeting for a few anxious moments.

Their leader denounced the AMA from the lectern in vigorous terms, "The A.M.A. does not stand for the American Medical Association—it stands for the American Murder Association!" Armed guards turned back members of other groups which sought to voice their dissatisfaction. The young intern vacated the platform, and presumably is chief of surgery at some hospital today, having learned that you can't fight the system.

Another dissident, Dr. Robert S. Mendelsohn, noted that in 1975, 787,000 women had hysterectomies, and that 1,700 of them died as a result of this surgery. He believes that half of these women could have been saved, as their surgery was needless. The *Washington Post* noted on January 21, 1988 that "Most heart pacemakers may be unneeded; more than half are not clearly beneficial." The story noted that one American in 500 now has a pacemaker. This business is only twenty years old, but there are now 120,000 implants each year, a business taking in one and a half billion dollars a year. Greenspan complained that "many internists are ordering them without consulting a heart specialist."

Dr. Mendelsohn has also complained that terramycin was an ineffective antibiotic, its major result being that it left children with yellow-greenish teeth and tetracyclin deposits in their bones. He quotes the Boston Collaborative Drug Surveillance Program, which found that the risk of being killed by drug therapy in an American hospital was one in a thousand, and that 30,000 Americans died each year from adverse reactions to drugs prescribed for them by their doctors. Mendelsohn minces no words in his opinion of modern medicine. He calls it the Church of Death, whose

Four Holy Waters are 1) immunizations; 2) fluoridated water; 3) intravenous fluids; and 4) silver nitrate. Mendelsohn dismisses all four as being "of questionable safety."

By the early 1940s, ranking members of the AMA had come to the conclusion that much of their problems with their membership lay with the abrasive Morris Fishbein. Most doctors were ultraconservative in their thinking, and they found Fishbein's antics repulsive. Nevertheless, he had spun his web at the AMA so fine that it involved everyone in the headquarters. His power was built on censorship, intimidation, and exercise of his powers to the limit.

It took his rivals almost a decade to get rid of him. Their opportunity came when Fishbein's able lieutenant, Dr. Olin West, became ill, and was no longer able to maintain iron control of the AMA headquarters for the Fishbein regime. Apparently ignorant of the cabal against him, Fishbein continued his merry life of travel and recreation, continuing to garner many awards and prizes for his medical public relations work. He had been named an Officer of the Cross in the exclusive order of Orange-Nassau, a very secretive organization which commemorated the invasion and takeover of England by William of Orange, and the subsequent establishment of the Bank of England. Fishbein made frequent trips to England, where he was wined and dined by prominent members of the Establishment; they must have believed he could be of use to them.

However, none of these honors proved to be of avail when the man who was described by *Newsweek* as "the man with one hundred enemies" (surely the understatement of the year), was thrown out even more unceremoniously than his predecessor, the unsavory quack, "Doc" Simmons. Despite repeated public criticisms of his junkets and abuse of his expense accounts, Fishbein confidently announced at a luncheon on June 4, 1949 that he would be around for at least five more years. He counted heavily on the traditional schism between two groups at the AMA, the liberals and the conservatives, whom Fishbein declared would never be able to agree on anything. He was wrong, because they did agree that he should be kicked out. United by their common hatred of Morris Fishbein, they formed their conspiracy to assassinate their Caesar. In describing this episode, Martin Mayer notes that since 1944, a sizeable faction at the AMA had been resolved to get Fishbein out at any cost. He had been exposed on a national radio program, Town Meeting of the Air, in early 1949, as a habitual liar. He claimed that he had been touring England, visiting the offices of general practitioners every day. The radio program revealed that he had actually been attending the Olympics, that he had dined with several members of the British aristocracy and attended a number of plays in London, and then had travelled to Paris for a round of the night clubs, all in the name of promoting medicine. The program, aired on February 22, 1949 by Nelson Cruikshank, demolished Fishbein's reputation, noting that Fishbein had not gone near any doctor's office in England during his stay. As for Fishbein's report about his trip, Cruikshank branded it a lie, calling it "a libel on a profession which is proud of its tradition of service to its patients. Fishbein's life was described as "a constant round of visits to New York plays, the Stork Club, and night clubs in London and Paris."

As a result of this publicity, the AMA at its 1949 convention passed a unanimous resolution that Dr. Morris Fishbein be removed from all posts in which he did any writing and speaking. This resolution provided that it be implemented "as soon as possible," which turned out to be that very afternoon. By evening, Fishbein was gone from AMA headquarters, never to return. One of the literary losses of Fishbein's departure was his column, which he had fancifully termed "Dr. Pepys Diary." It was described by one critic as "a running or logorrhic account of Morris Fishbein's private life. Each Christmas, the Diary was enshrined between boards and distributed as the Fishbein Christmas Card to nearly everyone who had a permanent mailing address." Like all of Fishbein's extravagances, the expense of this largesse was entirely borne by the dues-paying members of the AMA.

For years, Fishbein had used the awesome power of the AMA Seal of Acceptance to force drug companies to accede to his wishes. *Harper's Magazine* noted (Nov. 1949) that "The Seal is probably the biggest single 'puller' of advertising ever concocted. The *Journal* is far and away the most profitable publication in the world. Fishbein's absolute power—he often talked as if he carried the seal in his pocket—was also the source of other men's power."

After Fishbein's forced departure, AMA officials moved to dilute the center of power at the Chicago Headquarters. The Council on Pharmacy and Chemistry changed its name to the Council on Drugs in 1956; the Seal of Acceptance was dropped entirely. Ben Gaffin and Associates had reported to the AMA, "The advertisers, in general, feel that the AMA, especially through the Councils, distrusts them and views them as potential crooks who would become actively unethical if not constantly watched." This had been Fishbein's paranoid approach, but his attitude had been based on the need to maintain control and to force "contributions" from the ethical drug manufacturers." As soon as the Seal of Acceptance was dropped, AMA's revenues from advertisers doubled in five years; in ten years, it had tripled, from $4 million a year to over $12 million. In retrospect, Fishbein's arrogance and his shortsighted policies had been costing the AMA millions of dollars a year in lost revenues.

Dr. Ernest Howard of the AMA offered gratuitous reasons for dropping the Seal, saying "it was too arbitrary, and too much authority was vested in one body. there were also certain legal problems."

Despite the fact that Fishbein had gone, some aspects of his malign influence lingered at the AMA headquarters for years; costing the organization many million of dollars and a great deal of unfavorable publicity. Especially virulent was Fishbein's burning determination to destroy any possibility of "socialized medicine" in the United States. It was paradoxical that the AMA leadership under Fishbein's dominance should be so vehemently against "government intervention" in the medical field, when they had used government agencies for years for their own purposes, particularly the Food and Drug Administration, the U.S. Public Health Service, and the National Cancer Institute. One authority, James G. Burrow, traces the AMA's stance towards compulsory health insurance, which changed from exploratory interest to violent hostility between 1917 and 1920. This stance was justified as "anti-Communism," it being well known that Socialized Medicine had long been a primary goal of the Communist Party. A select group of prominent American leftists had been summoned to Moscow for special indoctrination in this goal. They attended a summer course at Moscow University on "the organization of medicine as a state function." The group included such stalwart liberals as George S. Counts and John Dewey. On their return, they began a campaign of public agitation for national health care. Their first convert was a "liberal Republican," Senator Henry Cabot Lodge. In fact, he represented the New England group of bankers who were allied with Rockefeller in maintaining the Medical Monopoly. On March 1, 1940, Senator Lodge introduced a bill for health insurance, which provided forty dollars a year for health care. The bill was quickly shelved, but the gauntlet had been thrown down. Fishbein had no intention of turning his fiefdom over to any government department. Over the next several decades, the AMA spent many millions of dollars fighting "socialized medicine," all of it raised by special levies on American doctors. It also became enmeshed in several expensive antitrust cases as a result of its activities.

As early as 1938, the AMA had been indicted by the Department of Justice in the Group Health Association case. In 1937, a group of government employees had borrowed $40 from Home Owners Loan Company to start a group hospital. The plan offered group medical care for $26 a year for an individual, or $39 a year for a family. This association, which took the name Group Health Association, hired nine physicians. The District of Columbia Medical Society then refused these physicians permission to use the hospitals or to consult specialists. On April 4, 1941, a jury found the AMA and the District Medical Society guilty of anti-trust law violations. The two organizations and eleven physicians had been indicted for restraint of trade. Those convicted included Dr. Morris Fishbein. Two and a half years later, the Supreme Court upheld their conviction in 1943. A fine of $2,500 was levied, and the AMA was ordered to cease and desist in its interference with the Group Health Association.

The AMA fared little better in its twenty year battle against Medicare. The preservation of the integrity of the local physician was a worthwhile goal; however, he was already under the control of the Rockefeller Medical Monopoly; it is difficult to see how the establishment of socialized medicine in the United States would change anything, nor has it. *Time* noted on December 10, 1948 that the AMA had assessed each of its members $25 for a campaign to spend $3½ million on ' 'medical education," a campaign to turn people against socialized medicine. It was the first such assessment of the AMA in its hundred years of operation. Almost two decades later, the *Saturday Evening Post* noted in its issue of January 1, 1966 that the AMA had spent five million dollars in 1964 and 1965 battling the medicare lobby in Washington. It was noted that the AMA had $23 million income that year from its annual dues of $45 per year, and from the sales of advertisements in AMA publications to drug companies and medical supply houses.

Time on Dec. 1, 1978 noted that Judge Fred Barnes, administrative law judge at the Federal Trade Commission, had ruled that the AMA Code of Ethics illegally restrains competition among doctors by preventing them from advertising. He further ruled that AMA ethical guidelines should in the future be approved by the FTC. The AMA issued an indignant press release opposing the decision; "There is no legal precedent in the United States for the federal bureaucracy to write or approve a code of ethics for any of the learned professions."

The subject of the AMA Code of Ethics had already come up several times. *Science* magazine noted on June 21, 1940 on "the bureau of investigation of frauds and charlatans" that the question was raised, "Should medical ethics be changed? The principle of medical ethics as set down at present, can be improved in wording and arrangement, but it also believes that the present is not the time to do the rewriting. It seems wise to let the muddied waters settle before any consideration is given to so fundamental nature of our organization as our principles of medical ethics." Although the speaker was not identified, this pious pronunciamento could only have come from Fishbein himself. The speaker goes on to admit, rather coyly, that "the principle of medical ethics can be improved" but that ended the matter.

The passage of Medicare, after the AMA had sent so many millions opposing it, apparently changed nothing. It proved to be an unexpected windfall for many of the more unscrupulous members of the medical profession. They had no problem in padding bills for fees to the tune of millions of dollars per year per practitioner. In 1982, Medicare paid out some $48.3 billion dollars, while Medicaid paid out $38.2 billion dollars. The more conservative estimates believe that some 11 billion dollars of these funds were skimmed in illegal profits. The heirs of Morris Fishbein at the AMA may have lost the battle to "stop socialized medicine" but they have won the war.

As we previously noted, the AMA trustees at a meeting on November 2, 1963, resolved to "eliminate chiropractic" their biggest rival, through a Committee on Quackery. The secretary of this committee reported back to the trustees on January 4, 1971 that "its prime mission, first, the containment of chiropractic, and ultimately, the elimination of chiropractic." A more blatant admission of conspiracy can hardly be found in any organization's records. The Committee's special investigative unit, headed by the general counsel of the AMA, Robert Throckmorton, involved using insurance companies, hospitals, state medical licensing boards, public and private colleges, and lobbyists. Every method of intimidation and censorship was used. Dr. Philip Weinstein, a California neurologist, had given many lectures to chiropractic groups on diagnosing illnesses of the spine; the AMA ordered him to stop all such appearances. He sent a note of apology after cancelling a forthcoming lecture, "Please accept our sincerest apologies for this late cancellation due to circumstances beyond our control. We were unaware that delivering medical lectures (to your organization) was prohibited."

Throckmorton also tried to put chiropractic schools out of business by preventing the government from granting guaranteed student loans or grants from the government for research at chiropractic colleges. He prevented them from getting accreditation; lobbied in every state to prevent the establishment of a government created accreditation body, and was furious when the HEW Office of Education, being an agency of educators rather than physicians, resisted his efforts and in 1974 sanctioned the Council on Chiropractic Education as a national accreditation body for chiropractic schools. The AMA brought pressure on C. W. Post University, a division of Long Island University, to drop a course designed for pre-chiropractic students in 1972.

In the late 1960s, the AMA Joint Commission on Accreditation of Hospitals imposed new requirements on hospitals; the AMA Principles of Medical Ethics barred its members from all forms of exchange with chiropractors. A JCAH letter August 13, 1973 to a hospital administrator declared that "Any arrangement you would make with chiropractors and your hospital would be unacceptable to the Joint Committee. This would be in violation of the Principles of Medical Ethics published by the AMA that is also a requirement of the JCAH." On January 9, 1973 the JCAH wrote to a hospital in Silver City, New Mexico, "This is in answer to your letter of December 18 referring to a bill which may be passed in New Mexico that hospitals must accept chiropractors as members of the medical staff. You are absolutely correct—the unfortunate results of this most ill-advised legislation mean that the Joint Committee could withdraw and refuse accreditation of the hospital that had chiropractors on its staff."

The AMA then forced the Veterans Administration to refuse payments to veterans for chiropractic services. These tactics had been reported to the AMA as positive results. A confidential memorandum dated September 21, 1967 by the Committee on Quackery boasted to the trustees that "Basically the committee's short range objectives for containing the cult of chiropractic, and any additional recognition it might achieve, revolves around four points: 1)

Doing everything within our power to see that chiropractic coverage under Title # 18 of the Medicare law is NOT obtained. 2) Doing everything within our power to see that registration, or a listing with the U.S. Office of Education, or the establishment of a Chiropractic Accrediting Agency, is NOT achieved. 3) To encourage continued separation of the two National Chiropractic Associations. 4) Encourage state medical societies to take the initiative in their state legislature with regard to legislation that might affect the practice of chiropractic."

Because of the flagrant activities of the AMA, several chiropractors finally sued, charging conspiracy. The case dragged on for years, and on August 27, 1987, after eleven years of continuous litigation, Federal Judge Susan Getzendammer of the U.S. District Court found the AMA, the American College of Surgeons, and the American College of Radiologists, guilty of conspiring to destroy the profession of chiropractic. During the proceedings, the AMA freely acknowledged that they never had, nor have, any knowledge of the content or quality of the courses taught in chiropractic college. Judge Getzendammer wrote a 101-page opinion, and issued an Order of Permanent Injunction requiring the AMA to cease and desist from "restricting, regulating or impeding or aiding and abetting others from restricting, regulating and impeding the freedom of any AMA member or any institution or hospital to make an individual decision as to whether or not the AMA member, institution or hospital shall professionally associate with chiropractors, chiropractic students or chiropractic institutions."

Thus ended the legacy of malice and obstructionism which Morris Fishbein had left to the AMA. Although he had been formally relieved of all duties at the 98th meeting of the AMA on June 20, 1949, the AMA had been bedeviled by his obsessions for four more decades. Another of his obsessions was his refusal to admit any black physicians as members of the AMA. He was often heard to refer contemptuously to "der schwartzers," a Yiddish term of contempt for blacks, whenever the subject of admitting blacks came up, as it did repeatedly during his regime. His policy continued at the AMA for two more decades, until 1968, when the AMA was forced to admit blacks. Previously, the blacks had maintained their own organization, the National Medical Association. In hailing the decision, *Time* referred patronizingly to "the moss-backed AMA."

The fact that Simmons and Fishbein were able to impose their petty concerns on this national organization for half of a century reflects little credit on its members. One of the most telling comments was made by T. Swann Hardy in the *Forum,* June 1929. In an article with the title "How Scientific Are Our Doctors?," Hardy wrote, "Medicine, as a profession, is not distinguished for the mentality of its members. The average intelligence is lower than in perhaps any other profession. Organized medicine in America is unalterably opposed to any standard of reorganization which would 1) make the medical monopoly thoroughly scientific; 2) make such therapy generally available to all who need it; 3) menace the incomes of incompetent practitioners."

It is noteworthy that the insignia of the medical profession is two snakes entwined on a staff. However, the University of Rochester, deciding that this was excessive, recently reduced the two snakes to one. The caduceus is the mythological symbol of the Roman god Mercury. He was the patron of messengers, but he also had a somewhat unsavory reputation as the associate of outlaws, merchants and thieves. In the ancient world, merchants were synonymous with the other two categories.

CHAPTER 3

THE PROFITS OF CANCER

In 400 B.C., Hippocrates assigned the name of Cancer or crab to a disease encountered during his time, because of its crab-like spread through the body. Its Greek name was "karkinos." In 164 A.D., the physician Galen in Rome used the name of "tumour" to describe this disease, from the Greek "tymbos" meaning a sepulchral mound, and the Latin tumore, "to swell." The disease could not have been very prevalent; it is not mentioned in the Bible, nor is it included in the ancient medical book of China, the Yellow Emperor's Classic of Internal Medicine. Unknown in most traditional societies, it spread with the rise of the Industrial Revolution. In the 1830s, cancer was responsible for two per cent of the deaths around Paris; cancer caused four per cent of deaths in the United States in 1900.

With the rise of cancer came "modern" methods of coping with it. A leading critic of the medical establishment, Dr. Robert S. Mendelsohn, comments that "Modern cancer surgery someday will be regarded with the same kind of horror that we now regard the use of leeches in George Washington's time." The surgery of which he spoke is the widely accepted and imposed method of cancer treatment now in vogue throughout the United States. It is called the "cut, slash and burn" technique. This method of cancer treatment actually represents the highwater mark of the German allopathic school of medicine in the United States. It relies almost exclusively on surgery, bleeding and heavy use of drugs, with the exotic addition of radium treatment. The Temple of the modern method of cancer treatment in the United States is the Memorial Sloan Kettering Cancer Institute in New York. Its high priests are the surgeons and researchers at this center.

Originally known as Memorial Hospital, this cancer establishment was presided over during its early years by two physicians who were stereotypes of the Hollywood caricatures of "the mad doctor." If Hollywood planned to make a movie about this hospital, they would be stymied by the fact that only the late Bela Lugosi would be appropriate to play not one, but each of these two doctors. The first of these "mad" doctors was Dr. J. Marion Sims.

Son of a South Carolina sheriff and tavern owner, Sims (1813-1883) was a nineteenth century "women's doctor." For years he dabbled in "experimental surgery" by performing experiments on slave women in the South. According to his biographer, these operations were "little short of murderous." When plantation owners refused to allow him to conduct further experiments on their slaves, he was forced to purchase a seventeen year old slave girl for $500. Within a few months he had performed some thirty operations on this unfortunate, a girl named Anarcha. Because there was no anesthesia at that time, he had to ask friends to hold Anarcha down while he performed his surgery. After one or two such experiences, they usually refused to have anything further to do with him. He continued to experiment on Anarcha for four years, and in 1853, he decided to move to New York. Whether his little negro hospital in South Carolina was surrounded by screaming villagers one night as they brandished torches, as in an old Frankenstein movie, is not known. However, his decision to move seems to have come rather suddenly. Dr. Sims bought a house on Madison Avenue, where he found a supporter in the heiress of the Phelps empire, Mrs. Melissa

Phelps Dodge. This family has continued to be prominent supporters of the present cancer center. With her financial assistance, Sims founded Women's Hospital, a 30 bed, all charity hospital which opened on May 1, 1855.

Like a later quack, "Doc" Simmons, Sims advertised himself as a women's specialist, particularly in "vesico-vaginal fistula," an abnormal passage between the bladder and the vagina. It is now known that this condition has always been "iatrogenic," that is, caused by the ministrations of doctors. In the 1870s, Sims began to specialize in the treatment of cancer. Rumors began to circulate in New York of barbarous operations being performed at Women's Hospital. The "mad doctor" was at it again. The trustees of the institution reported that "the lives of all the patients were being threatened by mysterious experiments." Dr. Sims was fired from Women's Hospital. However, because of his powerful financial supporters, he was soon reinstated. He was then contacted by members of the Astor family, whose fortune was founded on old John Jacob Astor's ties with the East India Company, the British Secret Intelligence Service, and the international opium trade. One of the Astors had recently died of cancer, and the family wished to establish a cancer hospital in New York. They first approached the trustees of Women's Hospital with an offer of a donation of $150,000 if they would turn it into a cancer hospital. Smarting from his recent firing, Sims double-crossed the trustees by private negotiations with the Astors. He persuaded them to back him in a new hospital, which he called the New York Cancer Hospital. It opened in 1884. Dr. Sims later went to Paris, where he attended the Empress Eugenie. He was later awarded the Order of Leopold from the King of the Belgians. Apparently he had lost none of his chutzpah. He returned to New York, where he died shortly before the opening of his new hospital.

In the 1890s, after receiving gifts from other benefactors, the hospital was renamed Memorial Hospital. In the mid-twentieth century, the names of Sloan and Kettering were added. Despite these names, this cancer center has for many years been a major appendage of the Rockefeller Medical Monopoly. During the 1930s, a block of land on the fashionable Upper East Side was donated by

the Rockefellers to build its new building. Rockefeller henchmen have dominated the board ever since the building was opened. In 1913, a group of doctors and laymen met in May at the Harvard Club in New York City to establish a national cancer organization. Not unnaturally, it was named the American Society for the Control of Cancer. Note that it was not called a society for the cure of cancer, or the prevention of cancer, nor have these ever been primary goals of this organization. 1913, of course, was a very significant year in American history. During that fateful year, President Woodrow Wilson signed the Federal Reserve Act, which was set up to provide funding for the forthcoming World War; a national progressive income tax, taken directly from Marx's Communist Manifesto of 1848, was imposed upon the American people; and legislatures had their constitutional duty of appointing Senators removed, they being henceforth elected by popular Senators; they all now had to compete for the popular vote. It was in this heady era of socialist planning that the cancer society originated. Naturally enough, it was funded by John D. Rockefeller, Jr. His attorneys, Debevoise and Plimpton, remained dominant in the administration of the new society throughout the 1920s. Its funding came from the Laura Spelman Rockefeller Foundation, and from J. P. Morgan.

From its inception, the American Cancer Society has followed the pattern set up by the American Cancer Society. ACS also had a board of trustees, a House of Delegates, and in the 1950s, it also established a Committee on Quackery.

This Committee later changed its name to the Committee on Unproven Methods of Cancer Management (note that it was called management, not cure), but the society still used to term "quackery" freely in referring to any methods not sanctioned by its trustees, or deviating from the "cut, slash and burn" method of cancer treatment.

In 1909, the railroad magnate, E. H. Harriman (whose fortune, like that of the Rockefellers, had been funded entirely with Rothschild money funnelled to him by Jacob Schiff of Kuhn, Loeb Co.) died of cancer. His family then formed the Harriman Research Institute. In 1917, the scion of the family, W. Averell Harriman, abruptly decided to go into politics, or rather, to manage our political parties from behind the scenes. The Institute was suddenly shut down. Its financial backing was then transferred to Memorial Hospital. The principal backer of the hospital at that time was James Douglas, (1837-1918). He was chairman of the Phelps Dodge Corporation, whose heiress in 1853, Melissa Phelps Dodge, had been the initial backer of what eventually became Memorial Hospital. She had married a dry goods merchant named William Dodge, who used the Phelps fortune to become a giant in copper production.

The Dictionary of National Biography describes James Douglas as "the dean of mining and metallurgical properties." He owned the richest copper mine in the world, the Copper Queen Lode. Born in Canada, he was the son of Dr. James Douglas, a surgeon who became head of the Quebec Lunatic Asylum. His son joined the Phelps-Dodge Company in 1910, later becoming its chairman. Because he had discovered extensive pitchblende deposits on his Western mining properties, he became fascinated with radium. In collaboration with the Bureau of Mines, a government agency which he, for all practical purposes, controlled, he founded the National Radium Institute. His personal physician was a Dr. James Ewing (1866-1943).

Douglas offered to give Memorial Hospital $100,000, but there were several conditions. One was that the hospital must hire Dr. Ewing as its chief pathologist; the second was that the hospital must commit itself to treating nothing but cancer, and that it would routinely use radium in its cancer treatments. The hospital accepted these conditions.

With Douglas' money behind him, Ewing soon became head of the entire hospital. Douglas was so convinced of the benefits of radium therapy that he used it frequently on his daughter, who was then dying of cancer; on his wife; and on himself, exposing his family to radium therapy for the most trivial ailments. Because of Douglas' prominence, the *New York Times* gave a great deal of publicity to the new radium treatment for cancer. The journalist headlined his story with a page one headline, "Radium Cure Free for All." The claim was made that "not one cents worth of radium will be for sale," Douglas was greatly annoyed by this statement, and on October 24, 1913, he had the *Times* run a correction. He was quoted as follows, "All this story about humanity and philanthropy is foolish. I want it understood that I shall do what I like with the radium that belongs to me." This was a rare glimpse of the true nature of the "philanthropist." His rivals in this field, Rockefeller and Carnegie, always give away their money with no strings attached. With this assurance, they were able to stealthily establish their secret power over the nation. Douglas had revealed the true nature of our "philanthropists."

The original press releases from Memorial Hospital had in fact intimated that the radium treatments would be free. They apparently believed that the great philanthropist James Douglas would donate his supply. The Memorial Hospital Rules and Regulations were immediately changed to stipulate that "an extra charge would be made for Radium Emanations used in the treatment of patients." In 1924, the Radium Department at Memorial Hospital gave $18,000 radium treatments to patients, for which it charged $70,000 its largest single source of income for that year.

Meanwhile, James Douglas, who had boasted that he would do what he liked with his radium, continued to give himself frequent treatments. A few weeks after the *New York Times* story in 1913, he died of aplastic anemia. Medical authorities now believe that he was but one of a number of personalities associated with the early development of radium who died from its effects, the most famous being Marie Curie, wife of its discoverer, and her daughter, Irene Joliot-Curie. By 1922, more than one hundred radiologists had died from X ray induced cancer.

Douglas' protege, Dr. Ewing, remained at Memorial Hospital several more years. He developed a number of ailments, the most annoying being tic doloreux, which made it embarrassing for him to meet or talk with anyone. He withdrew from the hospital, becoming a recluse on Long Island, where he finally died of cancer of the bladder in 1943.

Douglas' son and heir, Lewis Douglas, inherited one of the largest American fortunes of that time. He married Peggy Zinsser, daughter of a partner of J. P. Morgan Co. Peggy's two sisters also married well; one married John J. McCloy, who became the chief lawyer for the Rockefeller interests; the other married Konrad Adenauer, who became Chancellor of postwar Germany. Lewis Douglas became chairman of Mutual Life of New York, a Morgan controlled company. Early in World War II, he became a protege of W. Averell Harriman in the Lend Lease Administration. Douglas was then named chairman of the War Shipping Board, one of the famous "dollar a year" men of the Roosevelt administration. Later in the war, he succeeded Harriman as U.S. Ambassador to England. After Hitler's fall, Douglas was slated to become High Commissioner of

Germany, but he stepped aside to allow his brother-in-law, John J. McCloy, to take this post. The two Americans were pleasantly surprised when their brother-in-law, Konrad Adenauer, was named Chancellor. The family interests of the J. P. Morgan firm were firmly in control. In fact, Adenauer's earlier political activities in wartime Germany had centered around a small group of J. P. Morgan cohorts in Germany. They were ready to take over when Hitler died.

In the 1930s, two giants of the automotive industry were persuaded to become contributors to Memorial Hospital. Alfred P. Sloan had been president of General Motors for a number of years. He was also a director of J. P. Morgan Co. In 1938, he owned 750,000 shares of General Motors. He owned a 235 foot yacht which was valued at one and quarter million dollars in 1940.

Charles Kettering was an authentic inventive genius, responsible for much of todays auto ignition, lights, starters and other electrical systems. Fortune estimated in 1960 that Sloan was worth 200-400 million dollars, while Kettering was worth 100 to 200 million.

Alfred Sloan's credentials as a philanthropist were somewhat marred by his record at General Motors. He had steadfastly opposed the installation of safety glass in Chevrolet cars. During the 1920s, the lack of safety glass meant that a relatively minor auto accident, if it caused the breaking of the windshield or the windows of a car, could result in hideous disfigurement or death for the occupants.

Shards of flying glass would rip through the interior, slicing the passengers as it tore by. For a relatively minor amount, the ordinary glass used in automobiles during that period could be replaced with safety glass. Today, safety glass is required on all cars. Sloan made a public statement on this issue on August 13, 1929. "The advent of safety glass will result in both ourselves and our company absorbing a very considerable portion of the extra cost out of our profits. I feel that General Motors should not adopt safety glass for its cars and raise its prices even a part of what that extra cost should be." On August 15, 1932, Sloan again reiterated his opposition to the installation of safety glass in General Motors' automobiles. "It is not my responsibility to sell safety glass," he complained. "I would very much rather spend the same amount of money on improving our car in other ways because I think, from the standpoint of selfish business, it would be a very much better investment." The Alfred P. Sloan Foundation is doing well; in 1975 it had $252 million, which grew to $370 million by 1985. It and the Charles F. Kettering Foundation ($75 million) continue to be the chief benefactors of the Sloan Kettering Cancer Center. A liberal editor, Norman Cousins, heads the Kettering Foundation. The Alfred P. Sloan Foundation is headed by R. Manning Brown, Jr. Directors include Henry H. Fowler, former secretary of the Treasury, now a partner of Goldman Sachs Co., New York investment bankers—also director is Lloyd C. Elam, president of the nation's only black medical school, Meharry College in Nashville, Tennessee; Elam is also a director of the giant Merck medical firm; Kraft, South Central Bell Telephone, and the Nashville Bank; Franklin A. Long represents the necessary Rockefeller connection as a director of Exxon; he is also a director of United Technologies, Presidential Science Advisory Commission, professor of chemistry at Cornell since 1936, a Guggenheim fellow, he has received the Albert Einstein Peace Prize—he is a member of the American Pugwash Steering Committee, set up by the notoriously pro-communist financier Cyrus Eaton who was a Rockefeller protege—Pugwash is said to be directed by the KGB; Herbert E. Longenecker, president of Tulane University; he serves on the selection committee for Fulbright students, a very powerful position—his list of awards and honors in *Who's Who* goes on for several paragraphs; Cathleen

Morawetz, who is a director of National Cash Register, also a Guggenheim fellow; she is married to Herbert Morawetz, a chemist from Prague; Thomas Aquinas Murphy, president of General Motors for many years, also director of Pepsico, and the National Detroit Corporation; Ellmore E. Patterson, who had been with J. P. Morgan Company since 1935, he also serves as treasurer of Sloan-Kettering Cancer Center, and is director of Bethlehem Steel, Engelhard Hanovia, and Morgan Stanley; Laurance S. Rockefeller, who is director of Reader's Digest, National Geographic Society, and the Caneel Bay Plantation; Charles J. Scanlon, director of the GM Acceptance Corporation, Arab-American Bank of New York, and trustee of Roosevelt Hospital, New York; and Harold T. Shapiro, president of the University of Michigan, director of Dow Chemical Corporation, and Ford Motor Co., Burroughs, Kellogg, and the Bank of Canada—Shapiro has been on the advisory panel of the Central Intelligence Agency since 1984; he also is an advisor to the U.S. Treasury Department.

The governing board of Memorial Sloan Kettering Cancer Institute, called the Board of Managers, reads like a financial statement of the various Rockefeller holdings. Its principal director for many years was the late Lewis Lichtenstein Strauss, partner of Kuhn, Loeb Co., the Rothschild bankers in the United States.

Strauss listed himself in *Who's Who* as "financial advisor to the Messrs. Rockefeller." He was also a director of Studebaker, Polaroid, NBC, RCA, and held government posts as Secretary of Commerce and as head of the Atomic Energy Commission. For many years he funnelled Rockefeller funds into the notorious Communist front, the Institute of Pacific Relations. Strauss was also president of the Institute for Advanced Study, a Rockefeller think tank at Princeton, and financial director of the American Jewish

Committee, for which he raised the funds to publish the propaganda organ, *Commentary* magazine.

Another prominent director of Sloan Kettering was Dorothy Peabody Davison, a leading New York socialite for some fifty years. She had married F. Trubee Davison, son of Henry Pomeroy Davison, a Rockefeller relative who had been the right-hand man for J. P. Morgan. Davison was one of the group of five leading bankers who met with Senator Nelson Aldrich (his daughter married John D. Rockefeller, Jr.) at Jekyll Island in a secret conference to draft the Federal Reserve Act in November of 1910. The Dictionary of National Biography notes that Davison "soon won recognition from J. P. Morgan, frequently consulting with him, particularly during the monetary crisis of 1907 ... In association with Senator Aldrich, Paul M. Warburg, Frank A. Vanderlip and A. Piatt Andrew, he took part in drawing up the Jekyll Island report that led to the crystallization of sentiment resulting in the creation of the Federal Reserve System." As head of the Red Cross War Council during the First World War, Davison raised $370,000,000, of which a considerable number of millions were diverted to Russia to salvage the floundering Bolshevik government. His son and namesake, Henry P. Davison married Anne Stillman, daughter of James Stillman, head of the National City Bank which handled the enormous cash flow accruing to the Standard Oil Company. H. P. also became a partner of J. P. Morgan Co.; his brother, F. Trubee Davison, married Dorothy Peabody, the nation's leading philanthropic family. The Peabodys may be said to have invented the concept of foundation philanthropy, the first major foundation being the Peabody Education Fund, set up in 1865 by George Peabody, founder of the J. P. Morgan banking firm; it later became the Rockefeller Foundation. Dorothy Peabody's father was the renowned Endicott Peabody, founder of the Establishment training school, Groton, where Franklin D. Roosevelt and many other front men were educated.

Dorothy Peabody was on the national board of the American Cancer Society for many years, as well as director of Sloan Kettering. She was also a noted big game hunter, making many forays to India and Africa, and winning many trophies for her prize animals. Her husband was Secretary of War for air from 1926- 32, and was president of the American Museum of Natural History for many years; this was Theodore Roosevelt's favorite charity. Her son, Endicott Peabody Davison, became secretary to the J. P. Morgan Co., and then general manager of the London branch of the firm; he has been president of U.S. Trust since 1979, director of the defense firms Scovill Corporation and Todd Shipyards, also the Discount Corporation. He is a trustee of the Metropolitan Museum of Art and the Markle Foundation, which makes key grants in the communications media. Eisenhower's Secretary of State, John Foster Dulles, was also related to the Rockefellers through the Pomeroy family.

The present Board of Managers of Memorial Sloan Kettering Cancer Center include Edward J. Beattie, a Markle scholar at George Washington University, and staff member of Rockefeller Hospital since 1978, fellow of the American Cancer Society, and chief medical officer of Memorial since 1965; Peter O. Crisp, who is manager of investments for the Rockefeller Family Associates; Harold Fisher, chairman of Exxon Corp., the flag-bearer of the Rockefeller fortune; Clifton C. Garvin, Jr., president of Exxon Corporation, director of Citicorp, Citibank (the former National City Bank), Pepsico, J. C. Penney, TRW, Equitable Life, Corning Glass, and the drug firm Johnson and Johnson; Louis V. Gerstner, Jr., president of the giant Squibb drug firm, director of American Express, Caterpillar and Melville Corp.; he is a member of the visiting committee at Harvard University; Ellmore C. Patterson, with J. P. Morgan since 1935, married Anne Hyde Choate, of New York's leading legal family; Patterson is treasurer of Memorial Sloan

Kettering; he is also a trustee of Carnegie Endowment for International Peace, which was formerly headed by Alger Hiss; Patterson's brother-in-law, Arthur H. Choate, Jr. was a partner of J. P. Morgan Co. for some years; he then joined Clark Dodge & Co.; Robert V. Roosa, partner of the investment bankers Brown Brothers Harriman, a Rhodes Scholar who was the mastermind of the Federal Reserve System for many years, training Paul Volcker and then nominating him to be chairman of the Federal Reserve Board of Governors in Washington; Roosa also helped David Rockefeller set up the Trilateral Commission, of which he remains a director; Benno C. Schmidt, managing partner of the investment bankers J. H. Whitney Co. for many years, which has large holdings in Schlumberger, Freeport Minerals, and CBS; Schmidt was general counsel of the War Production Board during World War II, and managed the Office of Foreign Liquidation in 1945 and 1946, which disposed of billions of dollars worth of material at giveaway prices; Schmidt was on the President's Cancer Panel from 1971-80; he is a director of General Motors Cancer Research Foundation, Carnegie Endowment for International Peace, and the Whitney Museum; he received the Cleveland Award for distinguished service in the crusade for cancer control from the American Cancer Society in 1972 (these groups are always awarding each other honors and prizes, no one else need apply); Schmidt also received the Bristol Myers award for distinguished service in cancer research in 1979; his son, Benno Schmidt, Jr., married the boss' daughter, Helen Cushing Whitney, and is now president of Yale University; he had served as law clerk to Chief Justice Warren at the Supreme Court and later held the office of legal counsel to the Department of Justice.

Other members of the Board of Managers are H. Virgil Sherrill, president of the investment firm Bache Halsey Stuart Shields, which is now Prudential Bache; Frank Seitz, director of Organon, the Ogden Corp. both of which are chemical firms; he has been chairman of the key political group, the Institute for Strategic Studies since 1975; Seitz is on the board of the National Cancer Advisory Board and the Rockefeller Foundation; he also serves on the Belgian American Educational Foundation which was set up by Herbert Hoover after World War I to conceal his profits from his Belgian charitable work; Seitz also serves on the board of the John Simon Guggenheim Foundation which had assets of $105 million in 1985, and from which it spent only $7½ million in its charitable work; William S. Sneath, president of the giant chemical firm Union Carbide Corp., which has had several accidents in its chemical factories in recent years; he is also a director of Metropolitan Life, controlled by the Morgan interests, Rockwell International, and the giant advertising firm, JWT Group; Lewis Thomas, whose exploits take up a full column in *Who's Who;* he is investment counselor for the Rockefeller Institute, dean of the medical school at Yale, professor of medicine at Cornell since 1973; Thomas is a director of the drug firm Squibb, president emeritus of Memorial Sloan Kettering, director of the Rand Institute, Rockefeller University, John Simon Guggenheim Foundation, Menninger Foundation, Lounsbery Foundation, the Sidney Farber Cancer Institute, and the Aaron Diamond Foundation; J. S. Wickerham who is vice president of the Morgan bank, Morgan Guaranty Trust; Harper Woodward, who is with the Rockefeller Family Associates, longtime associate of Laurance Rockefeller.

This is only the Board of Managers of Memorial Sloan Kettering, the nation's preeminent cancer center. Each person on the Board of Managers shows many direct or indirect links with the Rockefeller interests. The Center's Board of Overseers includes Mrs. Elmer Bobst, widow of the prominent drug manufacturer and reorganizer of the American Cancer Society; Dr. James B. Fisk, chairman of Bell Telephone Laboratories, director of American

Cynanamid, Corning, Equitable Life, John Simon Guggenheim Foundation, Chase Manhattan Bank (the Rockefeller Bank), board of overseers at Harvard, and director of the Cabot Corporation; Richard M. Furlaud, chairman of the giant drug firm, Squibb, director and general counsel of Olin Corporation the huge munitions manufacturer, and director of American Express; Dr. Emanuel Rubin Piore, born in Wilno, Russia, headed the Special Weapons Group at the U.S. Navy 1942-46, head of the Navy Electronics Bureau 1948, director of research at IBM since 1956, professor at Rockefeller University, consultant to MIT and Harvard, director of Paul Revere Investors, director of Sloan Kettering since 1976; he received the Kaplan Award from Hebrew University; his wife Nora Kahn is a longstanding health analyst with the New York City Health Department since 1957, director of the Commonwealth Fund, Blue Cross Senior Fellow, United Hospital Fund, Robert Wood Johnson Foundation (of the drug firm Johnson and Johnson), Pew Memorial Trust, Vera Foundation, Urban League, grantee from U.S. Public Health Service; James D. Robinson III, chairman of American Express, which has now incorporated both Kuhn, Loeb Co. and Lehman Brothers investment banking houses into Shearson Lehman Hutton; he was formerly with Morgan Guaranty Trust, and is now director of Bristol Myers drug firm, Coca Cola, Fire-mans Fund Insurance, chairman of Memorial Sloan Kettering, and Rockefeller University; James S. Rockefeller, director of Cranston Print Works; Laurance Rockefeller, who is director of Reader's Digest with 18 million circulation and National Geographic with 10 million circulation—meaning that he influences 28 million middle class American homes each month— Dr. Ralph Moss, former public relations director of Memorial Sloan Kettering, noted that Reader's Digest is often a barometer of orthodox thinking on the cancer problem. The Rockefellers remain the most prominent contributors to Memorial Sloan Kettering; William Rockefeller is also an overseer—he is a partner of Shearson Sterling, lawyers for the Rockefeller interests; he is also a director of Cranston Print Works and Oneida Ltd.; T. F. Walkowicz, who serves with the Rockefeller Family Associates; he is chairman of National Aviation and Technology Corporation, CCI, Itek and Mitre Corporation, Safetrans Systems and Quotron Systems; Arthur B. Treman, Jr., managing director of Dillon Read investment bankers for many years.

Not only do the boards of Memorial Sloan Kettering have direct ties to the Rockefellers; they are also closely linked with defense industries, the CIA, and chemical and drug firms. It is no accident that they serve on the board of an institution whose recommendations on cancer treatment mean literally billions in profits to those who are in the right position to take advantage of them. And you thought this was a charitable organization! The fact is the Memorial Sloan Kettering and the American Cancer Society are the principal organizational functionaries, with the American Medical Association, of the Rockefeller Medical Monopoly. In 1944, the American Society for the Control of Cancer changed its name to American Cancer Society; it was then placed in the hands of two of the most notorious patent medicine hucksters in the United States, Albert Lasker and Elmer Bobst.

Albert Lasker, born in Freiburg, Germany (1880-1952) has been called "the father of modern advertising." He focused on easily remembered slogans and constant repetition to drill his messages into the heads of the American people. Like other successful hucksters memorialized in these pages, he began his career as a journalist. He was brought to this country by his parents, who settled in Galveston, Texas. His father, Morris Lasker, became a representative for Rothschild banking interests, and soon became the president of five banks in Texas. He lived in a luxurious mansion in Galveston, was a prominent grain and cotton dealer, and because of extensive interests in West Texas, he became known as "the godfather of the Panhandle." He died in 1916, leaving his son Albert as his executor. Needing cash to expand his advertising business, Albert Lasker hurriedly sold the lands at a bargain price, which in 1916, was not very much. His business acumen failed him here, because more than one billion dollars of oil was later discovered on those lands.

At the age of sixteen, Albert Lasker became a reporter on the *Galveston News;* he soon moved on to a better paying position in Dallas, on the *Dallas Morning News,* the largest newspaper in Texas. He soon found that the real money in the newspaper business was not in journalism, but in advertising, which brought in most of the revenue. Lasker went to Chicago, where he talked his way into a position with Lord and Thomas, the city's largest agency. He was only nineteen years old. Because he had agreed that his salary depended on how much business he could bring into the firm, he became a fanatical hustler. At the age of twenty-five, he had saved enough money, together with his family's money, to buy twenty-five per cent of the agency. At that time, he was earning one thousand dollars a week; the president of the United States was then paid ten thousand dollars a year. At the age of thirty, Lasker bought the entire agency. He went on to participate in some of the most memorable advertising campaigns in the history of the business. He built a three and a half million dollar estate in the exclusive suburb of Lake Forest, Mill Road Farm, a 480 acre spread with twenty- seven buildings, and a million dollar golf course which Bob Jones described as one of the three best golf courses in the United States. At the age of 42, he had arrived. The estate employed fifty workers, who kept six miles of hedges clipped each week. The French chateau in the center of all this luxury was more magnificent than anything built by his crusty neighbors, who viewed him with ill- disguised dislike. For years, he was the only Jewish resident, and he delighted in bruiting it about that he intended to leave the estate in his will as a Jewish community center.

Lasker was always very active in major Jewish organizations, serving on the American Jewish Committee and the powerful Anti- Defamation League. His sister Florine founded the National Council of Jewish Women and the Civil Liberties Committee in New York; another sister, Etta Rosensohn, was a passionate Zionist who headed the Hadassah Organization.

During the First World War, Lasker had been persuaded by his friend Bernard Barruch to join Woodrow Wilson's cabinet as an assistant secretary; this was to be his only government post. Despite the fact that he had built Lord and Thomas into a giant advertising agency, he felt that Chicago was too small for him; he soon moved his headquarters to New York. When he joined the agency, it had only $900,000 a year income, of which a third came from one product, Cascarets, a laxative. After he moved to New York, he realized that he was in a position to launch national campaigns to sell products whose stocks would then greatly increase in value. He cannily invested large sums in products which had not yet gained wide public acceptance, his most notable triumph being his promotion of Kotex. The press had long had a phobia about any mention of Kotex, and it was seldom advertised. Lasker bought a million dollars worth of International Cellulose, its manufacturer, and then launched a tremendous campaign in newspapers and magazines. He made many millions in profits on this one operation. Not only did he charge the firm for his advertising campaign, but he also reaped millions from the stock operation. He repeated this formula with other products, amassing a fortune of fifty million dollars. He later boasted that "No one has taken as much money out of advertising as I have."

Lasker was behind many of the nation's most successful radio shows. He auditioned Bob Hope, and launched him on a sixty year career. It was Lasker who made Amos and Andy the most popular radio show in the United States. He hired them for Pepsodent because he said that the half of the American population who listened to the show each evening would be envisioning the white teeth flashing "in those dusky countenances." The sponsor of the show was Pepsodent toothpaste. Although the program is now denigrated as offensive to American blacks, if Lasker were still alive, he would push it as the nation's most successful television show.

Lasker owned the Chicago Cubs, and was a heavy gambler. He was known to bet as much as $40,000 on a single golf match. He also was a hard driving taskmaster. In the depression year of 1931, he had a personal profit of one million dollars. This did not dissuade him from cutting back the expenses of his business. He took advantage of the widespread unemployment and the depression to fire fifty people from the staff of Lord and Thomas; those who remained had their salaries cut by fifty per cent.

One of Lasker's most successful promotions was his campaign to popularize drinking orange juice for the Sunkist company. He is best remembered, however, for his association with American Tobacco's George Washington Hill. When Lasker came onto the scene, Percival Hill was still the firm's president. The son of a prominent Philadelphia banker, he had built up a successful carpet business, which he sold, investing the proceeds in a tobacco company, Blackwell Tobacco; he then sold this firm to the tobacco king, James Duke. Duke reorganized the firm in 1911 and asked Hill to become president, his son, George Washington Hill, became vice president. Lasker got the account after World War I, when tobacco manufacturers were very conservative in their advertising expenditures.

They rarely spent large sums promoting a single brand, preferring to advertise their entire line. Lasker persuaded the Hills to concentrate their advertising, and to increase their budget.

They did so and sales skyrocketed. In a single year, Lasker increased their advertising budget from one million to twenty-five million dollars. He managed to maintain good relations with the arrogant and domineering George Washington Hill, whose crudeness was memorialized by Sidney Greenstreet in the film "The Hucksters." Greenstreet portrayed Hill as a loathsome slob who made his point by spitting a great gob on the table in front of his directors.

Lasker created the catchy slogan for Lucky Strikes, "It's Toasted." When World War II began, he tried to foist a supposedly patriotic slogan on the American public, "Lucky Strike Green Has Gone To War." The campaign was a flop. It was a flimsy pretext that the green color used in the package had been requisitioned for the war effort.

Lasker's greatest achievement was his national campaign to persuade women to smoke in public. He could be said to be the father of women's lung cancer. At that time, few women were bold enough to be seen smoking in public. Ably assisted by his minions in Hollywood, Lasker saw to it that in many scenes of movies, leading women would be seen smoking cigarettes in public. His greatest success was through Bette Davis, who delivered her lines in almost every scene through a thick cloud of smoke. Smoking in public now became common, creating a vast new market for cigarettes, which, of course, was Lasker's only goal. Some twenty years later, many of these women were dying from emphysema or lung cancer.

Lasker's furious pace took its toll. He had three nervous breakdowns, but his greatest shock came when his wife died in 1936. He met an actress the following year, Doris Kenyon, and impulsively married her. The marriage lasted only a few months. She went back to Hollywood, divorced him, and married the brother-in-law of pianist Arthur Rubinstein, which proved to be a successful marriage. In 1939, while lunching with Wild Bill Donovan at the "21 Club" who was soon to become head of the wartime OSS, later the CIA, he was introduced to an attractive divorcee, an art dealer named Mary Woodard. The daughter of a Wisconsin banker, she had started a dress company, Hollywood Patterns, designing inexpensive dresses for working girls, and then had gone into the art business. A few days later, while he was lunching with publisher Richard Simon, he met her a second time, and decided to marry her. He was just starting to build an art collection and knew very little about painting. He later claimed he had married her to save one million dollars in sales commissions, which he probably did. She tried to get him to relax, and soon had him going to a psychoanalyst. He was lunching with Richard Simon again when he jumped up and said, "I'm late for my psychoanalyst." Simon seemed puzzled, and Lasker explained, "I'm doing it to get rid of all the *hate* the advertising business has put into me." It is likely that he had put more hate in advertising business than it had put into him. Despite the fact that practically all of his close friends were prominent Jews, such as Bernard Baruch, Anna Rosenberg,

David Sarnoff, the New York publicist Ben Sonnenberg, and Lewis Strauss of Kuhn, Loeb Company, he rarely hired Jews in his advertising firm. When he was reproached for this, he merely smiled, and said, "Look, I went into this firm and took it over. Do you think I want somebody to do that to me?"

Among his proteges were very successful advertising men such as Emerson Foote, William Benton and Fairfax Cone, all of whom were gentiles. Lasker liked to call them his little goyim. He joked about how he could make them jump when he barked.

In 1942, Lasker, having made a large fortune, decided to close down Lord and Thomas. His proteges went on to found the firm of Fairfax Cone and Belding; William Edward, a lawyer, had married Carla, the daughter of Bernard Gimbel of the department store fortune. At the wedding, Lasker dourly cited an old Jewish proverb, "You can't make an omelet from two spoiled eggs." He was proven right; they got a divorce. His daughter, Mary, married the Chicago steel tycoon, Leigh Block, of Inland Steel. They amassed a multi- million dollar art collection. She also became a vice president of Foote, Cone and Belding. Block's brother Joseph became president of the Jewish Federation.

Lasker had grown bored with wearing white shirts; he started the vogue of wearing blue shirts in New York, which became the hallmark of the advertising profession. He never learned to drive a car, and had no mechanical skills. After moving to New York, he begrudged the enormous upkeep of his Lake Forest estate; in 1939 he donated it to the University of Chicago. The trustees promptly sold it off for building lots; the million dollar mansion went for $110,000.

Lasker's importance to this narrative is the fact that he and his cohort, a patent medicine huckster named Elmer Bobst, took the American Cancer Society, a moribund group in the early 1940s, and within months built it into a powerful national force. They used all their techniques for promotion, fund-raising and business organization to make this group the most powerful force in the new billion dollar world of cancer treatment, an achievement for which the Rockefeller Medical Monopoly was extremely grateful. They summarily dumped a cumbersome organization known as the Women's Army, which was very decentralized, and placed all the power of the American Cancer Society in New York. All of its meetings are held there. They also used their business connections to bring in a new board of trustees from the biggest names in banking and industry, charging $100,000 each for the privilege of serving on the board.

After launching the American Cancer Society as a viable organization, Lasker himself became ill with cancer. He was operated on for intestinal cancer in 1950, not knowing that cutting into a cancer immediately spreads it throughout the body. He died in 1952 at the Harkness Rockefeller Pavilion. Before his death, he had set up the Albert and Mary Lasker Foundation, which was to make Mary Lasker the most powerful woman in American medicine. She soon controlled a vast empire of grants, foundations, Washington lobbyists and other organizations. Her most able lieutenant in achieving this power was the Rockefeller employee, Anna Rosenberg, who has worked closely with her for years.

Elmer Bobst, who was Lasker's partner in putting the American Cancer Society over the top, was also a tycoon. Unlike Lasker, Bobst had come from a poor family, but he also had the born huckster's mentality, taken from that native American entrepreneur, P. T. Barnum, who said, "There's a sucker born every minute." Bobst joined the drug firm of Hoffman LaRoche in 1911, where his talents as a salesman got him the presidency of the firm. He was also a shrewd businessman; just after World War I, knowing that commodity prices were bound to fall, he was shocked to find that the firm had accumulated huge inventories in the New Jersey warehouse. He quickly closed a deal with Eastman Kodak to buy five tons of bromides, a key ingredient not only of analgesics but also of photographic supplies. He offered the bromides at sixty cents a pound, ten cents below the market price. Within a few weeks, the market price had fallen to sixteen cents a pound.

Bobst's great achievement at Hoffman LaRoche was his advertising campaign for vitamins. It was so successful that he won the nickname of "the Vitamin King." He made millions of dollars in the stock market, and he decided to leave Hoffman LaRoche for greener pastures. In 1944, he called in Cravath, Swaine and Moore, the lawyers for Kuhn, Loeb Company, to negotiate his terms; they got him a very favorable settlement of $150,000 the first year and $60,000 a year until his seventy-fifth birthday. Having made his fortune in peddling vitamins, he now moved on to the higher-priced pills, becoming head of Warner-Lambert. This firm's biggest product was Listerine. Gerald Lambert, no mean huckster himself, had built Lambert Pharmacal into a giant empire, principally through his relentless warnings about the perils of "bad breath." His father had invented a mouthwash, for which he appropriated the most famous name in medicine, Baron Joseph Lister, the inventor of antiseptics and asepsis in hospitals. A prominent surgeon, Baron Lister had operated on Queen Victoria herself, the only time she submitted to the knife. Gerald Lambert made his name a household word with fullpage advertisements for Listerine. Banner headlines warned that "Even your best friend won't tell you." Lambert coined a new word for this plague, halitosis, from the Latin for bad breath. At the height of the 1920s stock market boom, Gerald Lambert sold his firm to the Warner Corporation for $25 million, the equivalent of $500 million in 1980 dollars. The deal was closed in 1928; within a year, the value of the firm had dropped to $5 million.

The resulting Warner-Lambert Corporation had showed little growth during the 1930s. Bobst was hired primarily for his marketing skills, but he soon proved that he was an empire builder, buying more than fifty additional companies. In an astute move, he named Albert Driscoll president of the firm. Driscoll had just served seven years as Governor of New Jersey. As directors, Bobst brought in the shrewdest brains on Wall Street, Sidney Weinberg of Goldman Sachs, and Frederick Eberstadt, of Eberstadt and Company. As director of public relations, he brought in Anna Rosenberg, who had long been director of labor relations for the Rockefellers at their primary holding Rockefeller Center. This meant that Bobst had now established a key Rockefeller connection, as Anna Rosenberg continued to have a close association with her former employers.

Because he was the only one who was aware of his ambitious plans, Bobst had bought heavily into Warner-Lambert stock before he began his great expansion. As a result, the stock increased many times in value. He was now the largest stockholder, worth many millions. Fortune described his seigneurial life style, his vast estates in New Jersey, his 87 foot yacht at Spring Lake, and his suite at the Waldorf." In fact, Bobst owned five yachts in succession, each one larger than the last, and all named Alisa, the last being called Alisa V. He also married a second time, marrying the Lebanese delegate to the United Nations. He was chairman of the War Bond drive in New Jersey during World War II, and became a large contributor to political campaigns. He thus became a very influential behind the scenes figure in the Republican Party, so much so that he chose his own man for the Presidency.

Eisenhower's Secretary of the Treasury, George Humphrey, of the Rothschild Bank, National City Bank of Cleveland, had been slated to speak at a fund-raising rally in New Jersey of which Bobst was chairman. He became ill, and Vice President Richard Nixon was sent in his place. This began a close relationship between Bobst and Nixon, which was almost a father-son relationship. Nixon was dazzled by Bobst's millionaire life style, and he saw to it that the Bobsts were frequently invited to the White House dinners. In 1957, Nixon was able to introduce Bobst to the Queen of England at a White House gathering.

After Nixon's ill-advised, if justified, attack on the press after his campaign in California, it seemed that his political career was over. However, Bobst was not about to give up on such a potential ally. Nixon later fondly recalled the best advice Bobst ever gave him. Bobst had drawn him aside, during what was a period of great depression for Nixon, and earnestly told him, "Dick, it's time you learned the facts of life. You see, there are really only two kinds of people in the world, the eaters and the eaten. You just have to make up your mind which group you're going to be in."

At a time when Nixon had little or no prospects, Bobst went to his attorney, Matt Herold, the senior partner of the Wall Street firm of Mudge, Rose and Stern. Warner Lambert was their biggest client, and when Bobst "suggested" to Herold that he bring in Nixon from California as a partner of the firm, Herold was only too happy to oblige. With this springboard, Nixon was able to launch his successful campaign for the Presidency.

The move turned out to be a wise investment all around. After Nixon won the election, the Republican Governors of the states of New Jersey, Nebraska, Kentucky, and West Virginia turned over all of their tax-free bond business to Mudge Rose, giving the firm an additional million dollars a year of income. In January of 1971, Mudge Rose appeared before the Justice Department on the matter of the merger of Warner-Lambert and Parke-Davis, a decision which meant millions of dollars to Bobst. Attorney General John Mitchell, also a protege of Bobst, disqualified himself; his deputy Attorney General, Richard Kleindienst, then let the merger go through. These were the only deals which became a matter of public knowledge; no doubt there were many more. In a brilliant tax move, Mitchell advised Bobst to donate $11,000,000 to New York University for the Bobst Library.

In 1973, Bobst had his autobiography published by David McKay Company in New York. An obvious "puff" job, it was a glowing account of Bobst's accomplishments, unmarred by any unfavorable comments. When Bobst died in 1978, no obituary appeared in the *New York Times*. This was an amazing circumstance concerning one of New York's most prominent tycoons. The *Times* routinely memorialized even the minor executives of New York firms. Strangely enough, a public statement about Bobst did appear in the *Times,* a memorial eulogy by his longtime friend, Laurance Rockefeller, the chairman of Sloan Kettering. Rockefeller said, "His efforts in the fight against cancer earned the sincere gratitude of cancer patients and researchers as well as the general public." Perhaps Bobst's real memorial is the label of Listerine, which still carries the message, "For Bad Breath, insect bites, infectious dandruff; 26.9% alcohol."

Rockefeller was referring to Bobst's revitalization of the American Cancer Society. Under his leadership, it had obtained a new charter on June 23, 1944, and underwent a complete reorganization. The staff was expanded to 300, and the two hucksters launched a national campaign to enlist two and a half million "volunteers" to patrol every foot of the nation in gathering funds to "fight cancer." Because the orders to engage in this campaign always came from business tycoons, social leaders and politicians, the masses had no alternative; they had to obey. The huckster talents of Bobst and Lasker resulted in the often ludicrous spectacle of millions of peasants being herded out into the streets in an annual march to rattle tin cans and beg donations for the Super Rich. The only campaign to equal it probably was the annual drive by the Nazi Party in Germany for contributions for the Winterhilfe campaign. The ACS campaign operated on the same lines. The millions of "volunteers" threw themselves into this annual task because their jobs, their social position, and their families depended on their willingness to make the sacrifice to the God of Mammon, which was presently masquerading as "the Ghost of Cancers Past, and To Come."

The chairman of the American Cancer Society, Clarence D. Little, had been named to that post in 1929 by the Rockefellers, longtime associates who had established a laboratory for him at their summer home on Mt. Desert Island. He seemed to have no interest in cancer, spending most of his time as president of the American Birth Control League, the Euthanasia Society, and the Eugenics Society, the latter being a pet project of the Harriman family. He admitted that in 1943, the American Cancer Society spent nothing on research. Little had been president of the University of Michigan, and now served as Overseer of Harvard University. Under his leadership, the cancer group had been nothing more than a small group of elitists who met occasionally in New York.

Despite its reorganization on a more business like basis, the American Cancer Society, long after the Little's departure, continued to pile up a stunning record of nonaccomplishment. One critic, a longtime federal official, publicly stated that it should be called "the infantile society for national paralysis." However, the society's inability to find a cure for cancer was hardly accidental. The Bobst-Lasker influence brought it firmly into the orbit of the Sloan Kettering Institute, whose motto had long been "Millions for research, but not one cent for a cure." Charles McCabe, the irreverent columnist for the *San Francisco Chronicle*, wrote on September 27, 1971, "You might be wondering if the personnel of the American Cancer Society, or cancer research foundations, and other sainted organizations, are truly interested in a cure for cancer. Or whether they would like a problem which supports them to continue to exist."

The new Bobst-Lasker board of the American Cancer Society featured the usual array of Rockefeller cohorts, Anna Rosenberg, Eric Johnston, longtime head of the Chamber of Commerce and now head of the Motion Picture Association, a public relations spokesman for the Hollywood moguls; John Adams, a partner of Lazard Freres and head of Standard Brands; General William Donovan, the Wall Street lawyer who was selected by the British Intelligence Service to head the new Office of Strategic Services, the nation's spy network; he was later sent to Thailand as U.S. Ambassador to oversee the operations of the world dope ring; Emerson Foote, Lasker's advertising protege; Ralph Reed, the president of American Express Company; Harry von Elm, the super banker who was president of Manufacturers Trust; and Florence Mahoney, the multi-million dollar heiress of the Cox newspaper fortune, and a longtime crony of Mary Lasker.

In 1958, the officers of the American Cancer Society were Alfred P. Sloan, president; Monroe J. Rathbone, president of Standard Oil; Mrs. Anna Rosenberg Hoffman of the Rockefeller Foundation; General Donovan and Eric Johnston. Senator Ralph Yarborough of Texas, a perennial champion of socialized medicine, established a 26-member National Panel of Consultants on the Conquest of Cancer, chaired by Benno Schmidt, head of J. H. Whitney investment banking firm, other members were Laurance Rockefeller, Dr. Sidney Farber, former president of the American Cancer Society, G. Keith Funston, chairman of the Olin munitions firm, and Mathilde J. Krim, a former Zionist terrorist.

An interesting footnote to history is the revelation of the cozy relationships which developed between top Nazi officials and the founders of the Zionist terrorist network, Haganah and the Irgun Zvai Leumi, in the closing days of the Second World War. The Zionists were working to drive the British out of Palestine; the Nazis were also at war with England, which gave birth to the most curious political alliance of the twentieth century. One of the leading advocates of working with the Abwehr, German Intelligence, was one Yitzhak Shamir, now Premier of Israel. After the war, the Zionists employed many former Nazis to help set up their military opposition to the British. The leader in this alliance was the veteran of the old Stern Gang of terrorists, which was now the Irgun Zvai Leumi, none other than Menachem Begin. One of Begin's proteges was a young woman named Mathilde J., as she was known in terrorist circles. She was born in Switzerland after her father left Italy because of "poor economic conditions,"— no political ideology there. The present Mrs. Krim is described by *Current Biography* as a "geneticist" and a "philanthropist." She has been the resident biologist at the American Cancer Society for many years. In her younger days, she joined the Irgun Zvai Leumi, marrying a fellow terrorist in a show of solidarity. She soon became a favorite of Begin, and divorced her husband. It was Begin who was asked by a grinning Mike Wallace on the program "Sixty Minutes," "Did you really introduce terrorism into the politics of the Middle East?" Begin answered emphatically, "Not just the Middle East—the whole world." He was referring to the worldwide terrorist operations of Mossad, the Israeli Intelligence group which is entirely financed by the CIA with American taxpayers' funds.

Mathilde J. then went to work at the Weizmann Institute in Israel. One day, she was introduced to one of its wealthiest American directors, the movie mogul Arthur Krim. They were married, making her an American citizen. Krim has been the chief lobbyist in Washington for the major film companies for many years; he is also a principal fund raiser for the Zionist agitprop network. As a fund raiser, he was also a close friend of President Lyndon B. Johnson. Krim and his wife were house guests of Johnson's at the White House when the Israelis attacked the U.S. ship of the line, U.S.S. Liberty, killing many of her crew. When other American ships sent planes to aid the Liberty, immediate orders were sent from the White House for the planes to turn back. The Israelis were free to continue their attack for several more hours in a desperate attempt to sink the Liberty, to destroy the radio evidence it had gathered that the Israelis had started the Six-Day War. Although it is generally believed that Krim issued the orders for the U.S. planes to turn back, no investigation was ever made.

Johnson is now dead, and they are the only living witnesses in this horrendous example of high treason from the White House. The CIA had known for twenty-four hours that an attack was planned against the Liberty, in the hopes of bringing the U.S. into the war on the side of Israel; faked evidence had already been planted that the attack would come from the "Egyptians."

Mathilde Krim is now a director of the Rockefeller Foundation; she and her husband are directors of the Afro-American Institute.

Arthur Krim has a long record of supporting leftwing causes in New York, the New York School of Social Research, the Henry Street Settlement, and the Field Foundation. Krim is chairman of United Artists (now Orion Films). As personal attorney for Armand Hammer, whose claim to fame is that he was a friend of the blood soaked terrorist, Lenin, Krim is also a director of Hammer's two principal firms, Iowa Beef and Occidental Petroleum. Krim also served as chairman of the Democratic Finance Committee; he is chairman of the board of trustees of Columbia University, and director of the Lyndon B. Johnson Foundation.

Critics noted in 1976 that at least eighteen members of the American Cancer Society's Board of Directors were executive officers of banks. ACS spent $114 million that year, but had assets of $181 million. As of August 31, 1976, 42% of ACS cash and investments, some $75 million, was being held in banks with which these officers were affiliated. The 1975 budget of ACS reported that 570 went for administration; the amount allocated for research was less than the salaries of its 2,900 employees. The American Cancer Society for all practical purposes controlled the National Cancer Institute, a government agency. Former NCI director Frank J. Rauscher became the senior vice president of ACS, with his salary doubled to $75,000 a year. An ACS spokesman admitted that 70% of its 1976 research budget went to "individuals or institutions" with which its board members were affiliated. Pat McGrady, who served for twenty-five years as science editor of ACS, told writer Peter Chowka, "Medicine has become venal, second only to the law. The ACS slogan, control cancer with a checkup and a check. it's phony, because we are not controlling cancer. That slogan is the extent of the ACS scientific, medical and clinical savvy. Nobody in the science and medical departments there is capable of doing real science. They are wonderful professionals who know how to raise money. They don't know how to prevent cancer or cure patients; instead, they close the door to innovative ideas. ACS money goes to scientists who put on the best show to get grants or who have friends on the grant-giving panels."

This is probably the most reliable summation of what is done with your contributions to the American Cancer Society. As we pointed out earlier, it is the masses giving alms to the Big Rich, who know how to distribute these funds among themselves, their friends, and their favorite tax-exempt organizations, which in many cases are refuges for the more incompetent members of their families. The ACS directors are drawn from the "best people" in New

York, the jet set, the trendy Park Avenue crowd who were caricatured by novelist Tom Wolfe as "radical chic." At one time, Black Power was in; now it is homosexuality and cancer. This group constantly advertises itself as being obsessed with "compassion and caring," which is always done with other people's money. Their own wallets remain glued to their backsides. This is exemplified by the bleeding hearts on the national news shows, who nightly regale us with their version of the homeless, the starving in Africa, or wherever they can find a photogenic victim with flies crawling on him. These "journalists," who are paid millions of dollars a year, have never been known to toss their coins to these victims. In politics, its morals are exemplified by the fat, aging playboy, Senator Teddy Kennedy; in Hollywood, by the equally pudgy Elizabeth Taylor.

Mathilde Krim is now the guiding genius behind the newly created American Foundation for AIDS Research; because of her powerful Hollywood connections, she was easily able to persuade Elizabeth Taylor and other stars to raise millions for her pet project. She also recruited her old friend Mary Lasker as the first board member of AIDS. Mary Lasker paid the current "advertising genius," Jerry della Femina, to create a tasteful national ad campaign for the distribution and use of condoms.

The Memorial Sloan Kettering Cancer Center continues to be the most "fashionable" charity among the New York socialites; certainly it is the most influential. It is listed on the tony Upper East Side as the "The Society of Memorial Sloan Kettering Cancer Center." It has operated a popular thrift shop on Third Avenue for many years, which is filled with donations from wealthy families. Like many other young writers and artists, the present writer purchased his clothes there for years, all of it labelled from the most expensive shops in New York.

Because "the fight against cancer" is totally controlled by the Rockefeller Medical Monopoly, grants are routinely awarded which are nothing more than ripoffs. One wag claims the ACS will award a research grant only if the recipient signs a paper swearing he will not find a cure for cancer. Although only the tip of the iceberg has been revealed, there have been numerous exposes attesting that most of the "cancer research" is bogus, replete with faked results. In one of the more publicized incidents, the National Cancer Institute gave $980,000 to a researcher at Boston University, who was forced to resign after charges that he had falsified his research data; another well known incident at the august Memorial Center itself found that mice were painted different colors in order to "verify" certain cancer tests. Dr. William Summerlin of Sloan Kettering admitted painting the mice to make them look as though successful skin grafts had been done.

The National Bureau of Standards reports that half or more of the numerical data published by scientists in articles in the Journal is unusable because there is no evidence that the researchers accurately measured what they thought they were measuring. Alarmed by these statistics, officials instituted a survey; 31 authors of scientific reports were sent questionnaires asking for their raw data. The 21 who replied said that their data had been "lost" or "accidentally destroyed." What a loss to the research profession!

The reliability of the nation's researchers wilted under a blistering expose on "Sixty Minutes" on January 17, 1988, under the title, "The Facts Were Fiction." The subject of the expose was "one of the leading scientific scholars" in the nation. He had claimed to have done extensive research on the mentally retarded at a state institution, where the records clearly showed that he had only worked on goldfish. The "Sixty Minutes" report estimated that from ten to thirty per cent of all research projects carried out in the United States is totally faked, because of the requirements to win the "grantsmanship" race. "Startling" results must be claimed before serious consideration is given to requests for funding, which themselves are hardly niggardly amounts; they often amount to grants of millions of dollars. One scientific scholar who was interviewed on "Sixty Minutes" declared that "I would think twice before I believe what I read in the medical journals ... it is dishonest, fraudulent information." The moving spirit behind all this fakery is the unwillingness of the Big Rich to see their profits imperilled by any genuine advances in medicine. Therefore, the more fake research that is done, the less chance that a drug now on the market which is bringing in $100,000,000 a year or more will be knocked off the market. The wholesale fakery in American research is almost entirely due to the pressures of the Rockefeller Medical Monopoly and the drug firms under their control, who routinely present elaborately faked "tests" to the Food and Drug Administration to obtain approval for new products, concealing harmful side effects, which often include liver and kidney damage, or death. The control of the universities by the Medical Monopoly creates a breeding ground for more robotic minions, willing to abase themselves in any manner for a grant or a job which requires little or no performance. A lengthy history of faked research is an ideal "Panama" or control to keep these minions in line.

It is frightening to contemplate that such faked research is usually the basis for the acceptance or denial of new drugs, while protecting the Establishment as it continues to reap more profits from long outmoded and discredited panaceas and procedures. Yet this is the background, as well as the raison d'etre, for President Reagan's Brave New Budget for 1989, which sets aside $64.6 billion for "research and development." Although this is only a 4% increase over 1988, it represents a 52% increase since Reagan took office.

The National Institute of Health budget has doubled to $6.2 billion; cancer research will receive $1.5 billion, while AIDS is earmarked for an expenditure of $2 billion. Mathilde Krim must be very happy.

Critics have pointed out that Memorial Sloan Kettering had done practically no research on the prevention of cancer, only on its favored modes of "treatment." The basic premise of its researchers, that the cell is solely responsible for the multiplication of cancer cells, is probably erroneous; however, it is the basis for all of their work, including their promotion of chemotherapy. In fact, the cell is probably reacting to outside infection or pressures, and the fault is not in the cell. The Sloan Kettering approach dangles the promise of a "Magic Bullet," which will bring the cell back to a healthy regimen through medication, or chemotherapy. The chemotherapy drugs include alkylating agents which actually inhibit cell growth. They are alkaloids, which hinder cell mitosis or cell division. Sloan Kettering also bypasses the possibility of stimulating the immune system to respond to cancer growth, which is the normal method which the body uses to fight disease. This institution receives $70 million a year from various tax exempt foundations, including the Alfred P. Sloan Foundation, which means that the American taxpayer is subsidizing all of this research. One hundred and thirty fulltime scientists are doing research at the Center; all 345 physicians at the Center are also heavily involved in research. And what are the results of all this activity? A continued reliance on the now antiquated "cut, slash and burn" techniques still redolent of the "mad doctor" practices of the late Doctors J. Marvin Sims and James Ewing, dead these many years. While wedded to the ritual observance of these expensive, painful and futile procedures, the "Scientists" at Sloan Kettering maintain a resolute phalanx of opinion denouncing various wholistic procedures which rely on diet, nutrition and vitamins.

Dr. Muriel Shimkin of the National Institute of Health, wrote in the Institute's official primer on cancer in 1973 that "Treatment of cancer by diet alone is in the realm of quackery." Yet the American Cancer Society, faced with a growing amount of evidence to the contrary, issued a Special Report in 1984 advising the following program: "1. Avoid obesity. 2. Cut down total fat intake to 30% of total calories. 3. Eat more high fiber foods. 4. Eat foods rich in vitamins A and C. 5. Include cruciferous vegetables in the diet, greens, etc. 6. Be moderate in the consumption of alcohol. 7.

Moderate consumption of salt-cured, smoked and nitrite cured foods." This is a very sensible regimen; however, it has not been emphasized by the ACS or the NIH, nor do many doctors include this advice in their recommendations to their patients.

The American Cancer Society has always had one bugaboo, laetrile. Dr. Lewis Thomas, longtime head of Sloan Kettering, told the American Cancer Society Science Writers Seminar on April 2, 1975, "Laetrile had absolutely no value in combating cancer." This contradicted the work done by the Center's own scientists, whose real results had been suppressed. Dr. Thomas stated again in 1975, "Laetrile has been shown, after two years of tests, to be worthless in fighting cancer." Dr. Robert Good, president of Sloan Kettering had also stated in January 1974, "At this moment there is no evidence that laetrile has an effect on cancer." His own scientists had completed studies which showed the opposite; two researchers, Dr. Lloyd Schoen and Dr. Elizabeth Srockett, both working independently at the Center, had found that pineapple enzymes combined with Laetrile resulted in total tumor regression in 50% of their experiments on 34 experimental animals there.

One of the most famous beneficiaries of the laetrile treatment was the actor, Steve McQueen. He had been given up by his physicians as a terminal case when he tried laetrile. He was responding well until a physician persuaded him to undergo surgery on a tumor; he then died on the operating table of an embolism. The Establishment proclaimed that this proved the laetrile treatment was worthless.

Harold Manner, at the Cancer Center, also found a combination of laetrile, enzymes and vitamin A had a similar positive effect on mice with cancer. Dr. Kinematsu Suiguira, who had been at Memorial since 1917, after earlier working on cancer at the Harriman Institute, had also produced striking results proving that laetrile was effective on cancer in experimental animals. On June 13, 1973, the results of cancer tests using laetrile by Dr. Kinematsu Suiguira over a period of nine months stated, "The results clearly show that Amygdalin significantly inhibits the appearance of lung metastasis in mice." Although this had been announced by the Sloan Kettering Institute, on January 10, 1974, Dr. Robert Good, president of Sloan Kettering, denounced the news of the findings as "a premature leak." Dr. Ralph Moss, who was then public relations director at the Cancer Center, considered Suiguira's work a genuine breakthrough and a welcome departure from Sloan Kettering's singular lack of success in its cancer work. On November 17, 1977, he held a press conference at the Hilton Hotel in New York. Instead of receiving praise for publicizing the success at the Center, he was fired the next day. He later wrote an excellent book, "The Cancer Syndrome" which exposes many of the strange events at Sloan Kettering. His book is very factual, and is written without rancour against those who had thrown him out.

Because Elmer Bobst had played the crucial role in making it possible for Nixon to become president, he had little trouble in persuading Nixon to authorize a new and expensive "war on cancer." At Bobst's instigation, Nixon signed the National Cancer Act in 1971, which transformed the National Cancer Institute at Bethesda into a new monolithic government bureaucracy. During the next fifteen years, NCA was to spend more than ten billion dollars funding various cancer programs, none of which had any effect in curing or preventing cancer. In 1955, NCI had established a Chemotherapy National Service Center with a $25 million grant, to promote the use of chemotherapy. A fullpage advertisement in the *New York Times,* December 9, 1969, proclaimed that "Cancer Cure is Near at Hand." The story promised that a cancer cure by 1976 was a "distinct possibility." The chairman of the President's National Cancer panel submitted a report admitting that the first five years of the National Cancer Program was a failure; the cancer toll had risen during each year of its operation. By 1985, the annual toll was 485,000 victims.

More than 43,000 people deluged Nixon with demands that the NCI test laetrile. Benno Schmidt then chose a panel of scientists to make the tests; all of them were known to be fanatically opposed to laetrile. When he asked for the scientific results, he said, "I couldn't get anybody to show me his work." Had their tests shown laetrile to be worthless, they would have been only too happy to publish their findings. The battle against laetrile continued on a nationwide campaign. One lobbyist, Charles Ofso, had a fulltime job in Sacramento, California, lobbying against laetrile; he was paid $25,000 a year. Drug store proprietors who displayed books favorable to laetrile were informed that no member of the AMA would henceforth send them prescriptions until these books were removed. Since 1963, the Federal Trade Commission has brought pressure against publishers of pro-laetrile books. Government statutes not only prohibit the interstate shipment of laetrile, but even books which recommend it!

After chiropractic, laetrile was the most important target of the criminal syndicalist operation of the Coordinating

Conference of Health Information, the conspiracy launched by the American Cancer Society, the American Medical Association, and the Food and Drug Administration. It continued to be mostly a war of censorship and intimidation, whose goal was to prevent any public discussion of laetrile. TV shows which scheduled forums on laetrile, to discuss both sides of the controversy, were suddenly cancelled.

Tests showing the effectiveness of laetrile were suppressed; they never reached the public. The desperation of the campaign against laetrile was solely financial; it represented the greatest threat to the profits of the Rockefeller Medical Monopoly. Hospital treatment for cancer cost many thousands of dollars. Despite the Cancer Center's $70 million a year for "research," its Memorial Hospital charged $470 a day for a bed; a ten day stay would be nearly $5,000, with another $4,000 charged for treatment and physician care.

The record of the "cut, slash and burn" treatments were routinely distorted and falsified. Dr. Hardin James, professor of medical physics at the University of California at Berkeley, addressed the ACS Science Writers Conference in 1969; he revealed that the worst cancer cases were usually termed "inoperable" and deliberately left untreated. The published cancer studies of cures or remissions were the "sweetheart" cases, which had a high rate of recovery. Nevertheless, Dr. James reported, "the life expectancy of these untreated cases was actually greater than the life expectancy of those who were treated."

Despite Dr. James' revelations, the hospitals continued to pick and choose which cases of cancer they would treat; even the esteemed Cancer Center noted that its policy is not to accept some terminal cases; the patients are politely referred to a death hospice where they can die. In fact, such turnaways may have been a boon to the dying, as the treatment they would have undergone at Memorial Hospital would have made Count Dracula drool with envy. Dr. Ralph Moss revealed some of the prevalent surgical techniques there. He reported that cancer of the head and neck was treated by an operation called the "commando" after a combat technique used by commandoes in the Second World War; it called for the entire removal of the jaw. Pancreatic cancer was treated by removal of most of the area organs near the infected gland; the survival rate, despite this drastic treatment, remained the same, a mere three per cent. In 1948, Dr. Alex Brunschweig invented an operation called "total exenteration," which called for the removal of the rectum, stomach, bladder, liver, ureter, all internal reproductive organs, the pelvic floor and wall, pancreas, spleen, colon and many blood vessels. Dr. Brunschweig himself called this hollowing out technique "a brutal and cruel procedure," *(New York Times,* August 8, 1969).

The epitome of the "mad doctor" operations was known as a hemeocorporectomy. Originated by Dr. Theodore Miller at the Cancer Center, it involved cutting off everything below the pelvis. These techniques are more than reminiscent of certain procedures used by Communist revolutionaries in Latin America; the Sandinista revolutionaries were inspired by their leaders poetic dictum that "Liberty is not conquered with flowers, but with bullets, and that is why we use the VEST CUT, THE GOURD CUT, and the BLOOMERS CUT." In the vest cut, the victim's head was lopped off with a machete and his arms were severed at the shoulders; in the gourd cut, the victim had the top of his head lopped off; the bloomers cut called for hacking both legs off at the knees, leaving the victim to bleed to death.

The records of the "mad doctor" syndrome would fill several books. One special Congressional report followed some 31 "human guinea pig" experiments over a thirty year period. The Committee, chaired by Woodward D. Markey, D.Ma., gave his comment that his findings "shock the conscience and represent a black mark on the history of medical research." The report showed that from 1945 to 1947, in the Manhattan Project, scientists routinely injected eighteen patients with plutonium; from 1961 to 1965 at MIT, twenty elderly patients were injected with or fed radium or thorium. From 1946 to 1947 at the University of Rochester, six patients who had good kidneys were injected with uranium salts "to determine the concentration that might produce kidney injury"; from 1953 to 1957 at Massachusetts General Hospital in Boston, twelve patients were injected with uranium to determine the dosage that would cause kidney injury. From 1963 to 1971, 67 inmates of Oregon State Prison and 64 inmates of Washington State Prison had Xrays on their testes to determine the effect of radiation on human fertility.

From 1963 to 1965 at the National Reactor Test Station of the Atomic Energy Commission in Idaho, radioactive iodine was purposely released on seven separate occasions, and seven human subjects purposely drank milk from cows grazed on iodine contaminated land. From 1961 to 1963 at the University of Chicago and Argonne National Laboratory in Illinois, 102 human subjects were fed fallout from the Nevada test site, with radioactive simulated fallout particles, and solutions of radioactive cesium and strontium. During the late 1950s, twelve patients at Presbyterian and Montefiore Hospitals in New York were injected with radioactive calcium and strontium cancer particles. Oregon State Prison gave radium doses of 600 roentgens in single exposures on the reproductive organs, when the safe dose was 5 roentgens per year. For a decade, scientists were fed radioactive materials so that other scientists could calibrate their instruments for measuring these doses.

Whatever kicks the mad doctors may have gotten from these experiments, the cancer rate remained the same, or increased.

Congressman Wydner pointed out that "Information has been brought to my attention showing that twenty years ago, in 1957, the same proportion of cancer cases, one in three, was being cured. This raises the question why, despite all the money and effort devoted to cancer research ... the cure rate has remained the same." Despite such criticism, the NCI continued to waste billions of dollars on worthless programs. It was reported that George R. Pettit of the University of Arizona at Tempe had spent six years and $100,000 extricating chemicals from a quarter of a million butterflies as part of an NCI program; there were no identifiable results. Other researchers continued to find the war on cancer a profitable war.

The *Saturday Review* reported in its issue of December 2, 1961 that a prominent financial supporter of the American Cancer Society in Massachusetts was upset when he could never find the state director in his office. He was finally told that the director, James V. Lavin, was probably in his other office across the street, where he ran a private fund-raising company, the James C. Lavin Company; he represented a select group of clients. Stung by this revelation, the executive vice president of the American Cancer Society, Lane W. Adams, wrote a letter to *Saturday Review,* June 6, 1962 as follows: "The arrangement by which James C. Lavin operated private fund raising while serving as executive director of the Massachusetts American Cancer Society was known by the National Society." Adams said that Lavin's salary was $17,000, plus another ten thousand a year paid to his company. Saul Naglin of the Lavin Company was the controller of the Massachusetts branch of ACS for a number of years. The yearly overhead of the Massachusetts branch was $548,000 in 1960, with total income of $1.1 million.

Adam's letter also boasted that "We helped support the research of Dr. Sterling Schwartz injecting human leukemia brain extract in human subjects, Dr. Chester Southam injecting live cancer cells beneath the skin of human beings." Adams who had been with the American Cancer Society since 1948, now heads the national offices at 90 Park Avenue, in New York. He received the Albert Lasker Public Service Award from ACS; he is also vice president of Zion First National Bank in Salt Lake City, director of Paul Revere Investors, and the Energy Fund. Lavin's attorney, James Mountzos, was secretary of the Massachusetts ACS and also served on the national board.

In 1978, the American Cancer Society had $140 million income of which less than 30% was spent on cancer research, with 56% going to cover administrative costs. The Society had $200 million in investments. Before the Bobst-Lasker takeover in 1944, its income had never gone past $600,000 a year; the following year, it raised $5 million. In 1982, Allan Sonnenshein published a warning, "Watchout; the American Cancer Society May Be Hazardous To Your Health!" In 1955, in a power move, ACS took over all research from the National Research Council, executing a brilliant coup by creating a new Science Advisory Council to represent American hospitals and universities. Dr. Samuel Epstein, in his book, "The Politics of Cancer," noted that "apart from being uninvolved in cancer prevention, other than, to a limited extent, tobacco, senior (ACS) officials have developed for the society a reputation of being indifferent, if not actively hostile, to regulatory needs for the prevention of exposure to carcinogenic chemicals in the general environment and in the workplace." Epstein reported that the ACS opposed regulation of such potential carcinogens as Red Dye #2, TRIS, and DES. ACS refused to support the Clean Water Act, and blamed victims for cancer. EPA had reported that indoor pollutants cause six thousand cancer deaths a year and that 38 million Americans drink water with unsafe levels of lead and other toxic matter, including chlorine by-products. DES, diethylstilbestrol, was widely used from the 1940s to the early 1970s as a synthetic female hormone which was routinely prescribed by doctors to prevent miscarriage; it was not tested for possible side effects, nor did anyone know what they were. Finally, a student at the University of Chicago Medical Center showed that not only was it ineffective in preventing miscarriage, but it might have side effects. This finding failed to halt its use. In 1972, its longterm effects began to appear, cancer of the breast, with vaginal cancer in daughters of those patients treated with DES, as well as other genital malformations and abnormalities. It was also linked to liver damage.

Lee Edson, in "The Cancer Ripoff" notes that 74 private companies near the National Institute of Health in Bethesda were charging the government 144% overhead plus 9% profit to perform virus research. Nixon had placed his protege, Dr. Frank Rauscher, in charge of NCI; he was a virologist who began to promote chemotherapy as the answer to cancer. Dr. Rauscher claimed that the NCI chemotherapy program "has provided effective treatment for cancer patients all over this country, and the world." This claim was promptly challenged by Dean Burk, head of the cyclochemical section of the NCI, pointing out that "virtually all of the chemotherapeutic agents now approved by the FDA for use or testing in human cancer patients are highly toxic to markedly immuno-suppressive and highly carcinogenic in rats and mice, themselves producing cancers in a wide variety of body organs." Despite this criticism, Rauscher was then named head of the President's National Cancer Advisory Board.

The side effects of chemotherapy have been graphically described by many of its victims, the terrible nausea, loss of hair, sudden weight loss and many other adverse factors. A book by M. Morra, "Choices; Realistic Alternatives in

Cancer Treatment, Avon, 1980, reports favorably on all of the Establishment's cut, slash and burn techniques. Morra mentions diet only in its relation to nausea from chemotherapy; he soberly advises that you "let someone else do the cooking so that the smell of food won't nauseate you." Morra gave no advice on how to serve food without smell.

Since Memorial Sloan Kettering's first benefactor, James Ewing, dosed himself to death with radium in 1913, it has remained the treatment of choice at this Cancer Center. The *New York Times* noted July 4, 1979 that 70% of all cancer patients at Memorial receive radiation treatments, at a charge of $500,000 a year. It now performs 11,000 surgical procedures and 65,000 radium treatments a year. In 1980, Memorial bought all new equipment for its radium treatment, an expenditure of $4.5 million. However, radium treatment continues to be a horrifying treatment in its effects.

In 1937, Dr. Percy Furnivall, a prominent surgeon at London Hospital, diagnosed his own tumor as cancer. On February 26, 1938, he published in the *British Medical Journal* an impassioned plea as a result of his experience, "Tragedies from radium treatment are of frequent occurrence, and the publicity given to radium treatment of cancer is a disgrace to the Minister of Health and the vested interests which charge fantastic prices for this body-destroying substance. I do not wish my worst enemy the prolonged hell I have been through with radium neuritis and myalgia over six months . This account of my own case is a plea for a very careful consideration of all the factors before deciding which is the most suitable form of treatment." He died shortly thereafter, yet his plea had no effect on the continued use of radium treatments for cancer.

The late Senator Hubert Humphrey, who died of cancer, is often cited as an advertisement for radium treatment. Jane Brody in her *New York Times* book, "You Can Fight Cancer and Win," coauthored with American Cancer Society vice-president Holleb in 1977, cites Hubert Humphrey as "a famous beneficiary of modern radiotherapy." She glosses over the fact that "this famous beneficiary" was totally disillusioned with radium therapy before his death. In 1973 he was found to have cancer of the bladder; he was treated by X ray, and in 1976, his physician Dr. Dabney Jarman, triumphantly reported that "As far as we are concerned, the Senator is cured." *(New York Times,* October 6, 1976). Humphrey continued to wither away, undergoing more chemotherapy, until he flatly refused to go back to Memorial Cancer Center for more treatment.

Quoted in the *Daily News,* January 14, 1978, he called chemotherapy "bottled death."

The *Washington Post* in February 1988 ran a story "Cancer Treatment Toxic." "We are spared very little as we see healthy looking people turned before our eyes into shaking, shivering, nauseated bundles of misery. The successes, although few, have been dramatic."

One factor which has been consistently ignored in the development of cancer is the role of unusual stress. We all face daily stresses in our lives, with which we cope as best we can. However, unusual and prolonged stress places a greater strain on our system than we may be able to cope with. This is particularly true today, when sinister hidden forces poison all our communications with their shadowy propaganda, while assuring us that they stand only for "compassion and caring." A writer named Morley Roberts advanced a startling theory of cancer in 1926. An English scientist, Roberts belonged to no known school of thought, and because of his independence, his works have been largely ignored. His theory of Organic Materialism advances the following points:

"Malignancy and Evolution: Malignancy is the diversion of energy from high differentiation into the proliferation of low-grade epithelia which can endure irritation but only differentiate with difficulty." Epithelioma, a common form of cancer, is the multiplication of cells of the simplest type in the body, which, like those of the outer skin, the epidermis, are comparably short-lived and unable to differentiate. An organism afflicted with cancer is unable to differentiate to meet the conditions of its existence, because its energy has been diverted into multiplying low-grade cells. Cancer is the proliferation of low grade cell colonies in the organism. They migrate through the body seeking a place for themselves, although they have no function. Wherever they gather, they rob the higher grade cells of nourishment, where they are gathered into cell colonies as the organs of the body. These organs are choked off and starve, eventually causing the death of the organism. The modern State is a malignant organism dedicated to the proliferation of lower grade units at the expense of higher, more differentiated types. The more productive organisms are heavily taxed to support large numbers of nonproductive and poorly differentiated growths. The steadily increasing strain on the productive members of the State causes their premature death, just as the proliferation of the lower grade cells in the cancerous organism kills the higher differentiated cells. Roberts posits the question, "May we go further and even say that the common tendency to malignancy is the result of sociology refinements which ask for a higher role for epithelia?"

Morley Roberts posited a theory of the development of the organism, in which other cells began to gather around the execretory cell colonies of primitive organisms, and subsequently these cell colonies began to give off secretions which were poisonous to the organism. In self-defense, the organism threw up fortifications, or other cell colonies, around the vicious presence, which, in time, became part of the organism, and whose secretions became useful to it. Roberts calls this a theory of the development of the organs of the body.

The role of nutrition in cancer has yet to be seriously researched by the billion dollar boondoggles of the National Cancer Institute and the Rockefeller. Yet in 1887, an Albany, New York physician, Ephraim Cutter, M.D. wrote a book called "Diet in Cancer," in which he stated, "Cancer is a disease of nutrition."

Hippocrates coined the word diaitia, meaning "a way of life" which is what a diet is. In the classical world, "meat" meant the daily fare, and referred to oats, barley, rye, wheat, fruit and nuts.

The confusion as to the meaning of the word meat occurs in translations of the Bible. In Genesis, it is stated, "Behold, I have given you every herb bearing seed, which is upon the face of all the earth, and every tree, in the which is the fruit of a tree yielding seed; to you it shall be for meat." Hippocrates' advice to physicians was that they should first find out what food is given to a patient, and who gives it.

The ongoing controversy over laetrile revolves around the fact that it is a substance called a nitriloside. In 1952, Dr. Ernest A. Krebs, Jr., a biochemist, discovered that cancer is caused by a deficiency of nitrilosides, which occur naturally in over twelve hundred foods and plants. Animals usually instinctively seek out grasses and other plants which contain nitrilosides, yet when humans do the same thing they are attacked by federal agents. Some researchers believe that the adverse effects of carcinogens, radiation and sunburn on humans is caused by the fact that they are suffering from poor nutrition. These nutrition experts argue that coal tar does not cause cancer; and that the sun does not cause skin cancer.

Rather, these conditions arise from the sun's effect upon the skin of a person who is consuming too many sugars, fats and dairy products. The sun's rays create an acidic condition which causes these substances to rise to the surface of the skin, causing an irritation which can then become catalyst. It is noted that people in tropical countries, who are exposed to strong sunlight, rarely get skin cancer because they eat little meat and fats. It was also discovered after the atomic bombing of Japanese civilians that those who were still eating their traditional diet of brown rice, sea salt and miso vegetables, were little damaged by the same amount of atomic radiation which killed those who were eating a more modern diet of fats and meat.

Some experts note that they can detect cancer by the peculiar smell of a person in its early stages, the smell of decomposition. Others note that cancer can be detected by a greenish cast to the skin. The epidemic of prostate cancer among American men seems to be the result of a diet of rich foods, with frequent ingestion of eggs, meat and dairy products, and baked goods made with refined flour. A suggested remedy is a diet of fruit and rice, the same diet which is recommended to lower blood pressure and which has been featured at Duke University for many years. Beef is said to be particularly dangerous for prostate and colon cancer. Nutritionists believe that cancer represents a reverse evolutionary process, in which cells decompose or change back to a more primordial vegetable type of life. This corresponds in some ways with the theories of Morley Roberts.

It is notable that only four percent of the nations medical schools offer a course in nutrition. This reflects the

Rockefeller Medical Monopoly's obsession with drugs and its commitment to the allopathic school of medicine, as opposed to homeopathic or holistic medicine.

Nobel Prize winner James Watson declared at a cancer symposium at MIT that "the American public has been sold a nasty bill of goods about cancer ... a soporific orgy," as reported in the *New York Times* March 9, 1975. In January of 1975, Dr. Charles C. Edwards, a researcher, wrote to the Secretary of HEW that the war on cancer was politically motivated and was based on spending money. The prominent French oncologist, Dr. Lucien Israel, said, "Radium is an unproven method in many cases. indeed, there have been no conclusive trials" on radiation therapy. Israel terms it "a palliative for relief of pain, etc., temporary in nature." He also points out that "the medical community has been thrown into confusion by recent studies which have shown that metastases may be more frequent in cases that have received radiation." In short, the radiation increases the spread of cancer. It has long been known that cutting into a tumor causes it to spread throughout the body. The exploratory operation to see if you have cancer usually guarantees that it will be fatal.

Nevertheless, the American Cancer Society continues to back all of the losing methods of treating cancer. For twenty years, it has patently repeated its famous Cancer's Seven Warning Signals, which ignore chemicals in the environment and discounts FDA warnings about coal tar and hair dyes. In 1976, the ACS released a press communication, "Urgent Message; Mammography; Benefits and Risks." Dr. John Bailar of the Harvard School of Public Health, and editor of the prestigious NCI Cancer Journal, was horrified. He wrote a letter to the acting director of the NCI, Dr. Guy Newell, "I have just become aware of a problem that has the seeds of a major disaster. The Urgent Message itself is plain hog-wash, the statement is seriously faulty, and hence represents a grave danger to that bulk of women who should avoid mammography. " Nevertheless, the ACS flyer went to every hospital in New York, and to 15,000 physicians. Despite the known risks of exposing women to repeated X rays, the ACS still emphasizes annual mammographies as one of its most vaunted techniques for "controlling" cancer. Jane Brody's book, "You Can Fight Cancer and Win," recommends this and many other ACS goals.

The American Cancer Society also stands firmly behind radical mastectomy, the total removal of the breast in cases of women's breast cancer. This technique is frowned upon as unusually brutal and ineffective; it has long been abandoned in most European countries, including England, France and the Scandinavian countries and neighboring Canada. In 1975, when Rose Kuttner published her definitive work, "Breast Cancer" which was critical of radical mastectomy, the ACS refused to list or recommend it.

It was Elmer Bobst's goal to make the National Cancer Institute "autonomous," much as the Federal Reserve System is "autonomous." He was able to achieve this goal because of his longstanding personal connection with President Richard Nixon. As the mastermind of the American Cancer Society, he really intended it to become "autonomous" from Washington influence, while making it completely subservient to the American Cancer Society from New York. Rep. David Obey, Democrat, Wisconsin, noted that "the American Cancer Society wants to keep the National Cancer Institute strong in bankroll and weak in staff so that it can direct its spending without too much interference." A very astute observation. One of its directors, is Mary Lasker, who, thirty-six years after Albeit Lasker's death, is still described by Washington observers as the most powerful woman in American medicine. The National Institute of Health bought the Visitation Convent in Bethesda from the Catholic Church for $4.4 million; it now houses the Mary Lasker Center. Through her access to funding, the ACS maintains fulltime lobbyists in Washington, headed by Col. Luke Quinn, and aided by Mike Gorman. The Pharmaceutical Manufacturers Association, with Washington lobbyist Lloyd Cutler, also works with Mary Lasker.

Whatever else may be said of the American Cancer Society, there can be no doubt that it remains well insulated against reality. A leading Washington reporter, Daniel S. Greenberg, wrote in the *Columbia Journalism Review* in 1975 that cancer rates for most types of cancer had been static since the 1950s; some rates actually declined, probably because the use of toxic chemotherapy increased the death rate. One researcher told Greenberg there had been little improvement since 1945. Dr. Frank Rauscher challenged Greenberg at the 1975 ACS Science Writers Seminar, claiming that these figures were out of date; however, when the new figures were released, they upheld Greenberg's findings. This rings hollowly against the annual promises of "breakthroughs" when the two and a half million "volunteers" swarm across America shaking their tincans and begging for the rich. They have been making these same promises and raising the same amounts of money, or more, for almost fifty years. Laurance Rockefeller noted in *Reader's Digest,* February 1957 an exultant comment, "There is, for the first time, a scent of ultimate victory in the air," as he described "progress against cancer." Sloan Kettering director C. P. Dusty Rhodes was quoted in the Denver Post, October 3, 1953, "I am convinced that in the next decade, or maybe more, we will have a chemical as effective against cancer as sulfaniolmides and penicillin are against bacterial infection." Well, maybe more. In 1956, Dr. Wendell F. Stanley, a Nobel Prize Winner, reported in an address to the annual AMA convention, "Viruses are the prime cause of most types of cancer." Nothing more has been heard on this subject in thirty years.

One physician, Dr. Cecil Pitard, was informed that he had terminal cancer and that he had only a few weeks to live. The Knoxville, Tennessee physician was diagnosed at the Mayo Clinic as having lymphoma. Lymphatic cancer results because the body is no longer able to detoxify or cleanse itself. Tonsillectomies often initiate a deterioration of the lymphatic system, resulting in lymph gland inflammation, and eventually, lymphatic cancer. With nothing to lose, Dr. Pitard experimented on himself with the anti-flu bacterial antigen, staphage lysate and sodium butyrate, a fatty acid food found in milk and butter. He soon found that he had been completely cured. Nevertheless, the Cancer Establishment ignored his report, and became even more vociferous in its campaign against "unproven remedies." In most cases like Dr. Pitard's the cancer profiteers sneer that it probably was misdiagnosed and he never had cancer, or that he had a "spontaneous remission," which is their most oft repeated response. It would seem that they would show some interest in how to obtain a "spontaneous remission," because they have now been talking about it for half a century, yet we have heard nothing from the $70 million a year research program at Sloan Kettering about spontaneous remission.

After Dr. Ralph Moss had been fired from Sloan Kettering for revealing the positive results of laetrile experiments, he made public the fact that the Institute was sitting on many other results of successful treatment of cancer, including more than one thousand positive cases of response to the Coley treatment since 1906. Moss reported that Dr. James Ewing, "Coley's nemesis and arch rival, turned Memorial Hospital into a medical branch of the radium trust." Dr. William E. Koch, professor of physiology at Detroit Medical College and the University of Michigan, presaged freeradical pathology treatment with the development of Glyoxylide, which stimulated the body to oxidate toxins. Although his treatment was never scientifically refuted, Koch, who began oxidation studies in 1915 and used this treatment since 1918, was persecuted for sixteen years by the Medical Monopoly. He was finally driven out of the country, and died in Brazil in 1967. The FDA had started to harass him in 1920; the Wayne County Medical Society formed a "Cancer Committee" of doctors in 1923 who condemned Koch's treatment. His stimulation of cell oxidation treatment is by carefully planned diet which cleansed the system, yet this proven treatment is still denounced today by the cancer profiteers as "quackery." Koch tried to continue his work in Mexico and Brazil, but the FDA refused to abandon their pursuit. He was prosecuted in 1942 and 1946; the FDA finally obtained a permanent junction against the Koch treatment in 1950. Several physicians who had successfully treated cancer with the Koch treatment were expelled from the medical society. It was still allowable to kill a patient, but it was unforgivable to cure him.

Another independent physician, Dr. Max Gerson, discovered that a vegetarian diet, with raw fruits and vegetables, and no salt, cured migraine and lupus. He continued his studies until he found that detoxification of the body could cure cancer. In 1958, he published his findings in his book, "A Cancer Therapy," emphasizing a low fat diet, no salt and a minimum of protein. In 1964, he was invited to testify before a Senate Subcommittee, which produced a 227 page report, document number 89471. The copies of this report were never distributed by the Senate; it received no coverage in medical journals, and Dr. Gerson never received one cent from any charitable organization such as the American Cancer Society to either prove or disprove his findings, even though these groups claimed they were "researching" a cure for cancer.

Another famous case was that of Harry Hoxsey, who used a herbal treatment, based upon Indian remedies, for cancer for thirty- five years. In a well-publicized court battle, Hoxsey won a libel suit against Morris Fishbein; the good doctor was forced to admit under cross examination that he, the most famous doctor in the United States, had never practiced medicine one day in his life.

Dr. Robert E. Lincoln discovered the bacterioplage method of conquering cancer, in which viruses parasitically attach and destroy specific bacteria. He received national attention when he cured the son of Senator Charles Tobey with this method. Tobey was astounded to learn that Dr. Lincoln has been expelled from the Massachusetts Medical Society because he was curing people of cancer. He conducted a Congressional investigation, in which his special counsel from the Department of Justice, Benedict Fitzgerald, wrote, April 28, 1953, "The alleged machinations of Dr. J. J. Moore (for the past ten years the treasurer of American Medical Association) could involve the AMA and others in a conspiracy of alarming proportions. behind and over all this is the weirdest conglomeration of corrupt motives, intrigues, selfishness, jealousy, obstruction and conspiracy I have ever seen. My investigation to date should convince this Committee that a conspiracy does exist to stop the free flow and use of drugs in interstate commerce which allegedly (have) solid therapeutic value. Public and private funds have been thrown around like confetti at a country fair to close up and destroy clinics, hospitals and science research laboratories which do not conform to the viewpoint of medical associations.

How long will the American people take this?"

Thirty-five years, they are still taking it. The outcome of the Tobey Hearings is instructive. Senator Tobey died suddenly of a heart attack, as happens in Washington when a politician treads on dangerous ground. He was succeeded on the Committee by Senator John Bricker of Ohio. Bricker, for many years, was considered to be a dedicated conservative by millions of Americans. In reality, he was the lawyer for a number of large drug manufacturers and bankers, the ultimate establishment figure. He promptly fired Special Counsel Benedict Fitzgerald; the Hearings were then closed down.

Dr. Robert Lincoln was bold enough to sue the Massachusetts Medical Society for libel; he also died before the case could come to trial.

Dr. Andrew C. Ivy, vice president of the University of Illinois, began to use a preparation which he called Krebiozen. He succeeded in curing cancer with it; the AMA promptly published a report on Krebiozen which ruled that it was "of no benefit." A 289 day trial resulted, in which Dr. Ivy was cleared of all counts against him. Dr. Peter de Marco, a graduate of Hahnemann Medical School, successfully treated over 800 patients with PVY, procaine polyvinyl pyrrolidone; his license to practice medicine in New Jersey was revoked.

A favorite recommendation of the American Cancer Society is the "Pap" test for cancer, despite its many drawbacks. *Insight* magazine, January 11, 1988, criticized many diagnostic laboratories for doing sloppy work, quoting the *Wall Street Journal* of November 1987 that "Pap smears have a false negative rate of from 20-40%; a false negative means death by cancer." Stung by this exposure of a method which the ACS had frenetically promoted for many years, Dr. Harmon J. Eyre, president of the American Cancer Society, called a joint press conference of the ACS, the AMA, and the NCI, to renew their joint recommendation that all women from 20 to 60 have an annual Pap smear. At this press conference reported by AP, January 20, 1988, Eyre was quoted, "A main reason for calling the press conference was an attempt to counter confusion about the value of the

Pap test in light of recent publicity about the percentage of false negative results from some labs." Although he went on record with unqualified endorsements of the Pap tests, Eyre offered no answer to the problem of false negative reports or the terrible threat which it posed to many women.

Some women's groups are becoming alerted to the fact that the Medical Monopoly is needlessly condemning many women to death. The *Washington Post* noted, February 16, 1988, a report of a Women's Health Trial, in which 300 women demanded low fat tests in which fat in the diet would be reduced from 40% to 20%, the purpose being to diminish breast cancer. They asked for funding from the NCI, but the Board of Scientific Counselors of NCI refused to advance any funding for the project. The women's spokesman pointed out that "NCI is committed to breast cancer control rather than prevention."

What would the most powerful woman in American medicine have said about this? Mary Lasker has been content to play the part of the gracious Lady Bountiful with the money her husband earned as the nation's most famous huckster. At the American Cancer Society's Science Writers Seminars, which are held each year in some exotic hotel during the harsh winter months, *Science* noted May 18, 1973, that these spring seminars, held annually since 1949, always are held in warm climates, free junkets for science editors at big circulation newspapers and magazines. *Science* pointed out that these seminars, which cost ACS about $25,000, generate about 300 favorable news stories and result in ACS raising about $85 million in extra donations. This is probably one of the best investments around. In 1957, novelist Han Suyin, wearing an exquisite fur coat, delivered an enthusiastic report to the *Science* writers about how much good the chemical manufacturers have done for the health of our citizens. In all fairness to Han, Love Canal had not been discovered in 1957. The seminar met recently (1973) at the fabulous Rio Rico Inn near Tucson, Arizona. Not only are all expenses paid for the complaisant writers, but an extra treat, a Happy Hour at the bar at the end of each "work day," makes certain that the journalists float in to dinner in a very jovial mood. The Happy Hour is paid for by the gracious Mary Lasker. *Saturday Review* noted April 10, 1965, the ACS had an unusually effective public relations department. The secret of public relations is to obtain free space in major publications, instead of buying advertising. The Lasker connection also ensures that major New York agencies such as McCann Erickson, prepare advertising campaigns for ACS at no charge.

It is ironic that Albert Lasker, the co-creator of the American Cancer Society as we know it, and its subsidiary creature, the National Cancer Institute, should have built much of his fortune on his promotion of cigarette smoking. After his death from cancer, the American Cancer Society reluctantly came to the conclusion that "smoking is bad for your health." The mounting death toll from lung cancer forced the cigarette companies to consider alternatives; one of these was filters. On January 1, 1954, Kent cigarettes released an ad to 80 newspapers that AMA tests had proved the Kent filters were the most efficient in removing cigarette tar. Because this "proof was on a par with most other AMA claims, the AMA was compelled to protest to Lorillard, the manufacturer. *Time* magazine commented, April 12, 1954, "The usually soporific AMA barred advertisements for Kent cigarettes." When the Surgeon General released his 1964 report on the harmful effects of cigarette smoking, it panicked the industry, even though it had long been heralded by previous studies. In June, 1954, Dr. Daniel Horn and Edward Cuyler Hammond presented a report to the AMA convention, linking smoking and lung cancer. Horn and Hammond headed the statistical department at the ACS. American Tobacco, one of Lasker's principal holdings, dropped five points in one day after this presentation. Hammond was a well known epidemiologist who had served as a consultant to NIH, the U.S. Navy, USAF and the Brookhaven Lab. He was a vice president of ACS and director of its research. Although he had conducted extensive research on the effects of smoking, he steadfastly refused to share this material with other organizations. In 1971, he received an invitation to join a panel of scientists to discuss smoking; he refused, stating that it had been the policy of ACS since 1952 not to share data with other researchers. *Current Biography* reported in 1957 that Hammond smoked four packs of cigarettes a day; his wife smoked three packs a day They both died of lung cancer.

Despite the ACS revelations, the tobacco interests, which were closely linked to the Rockefeller Medical Monopoly, fought a determined rearguard action against the lung cancer campaign. One of Washington's best connected lobbyists, Patricia Firestone Chatham, widow of Representative R. T. Chatham, the chairman of Chatham Mills textile firm, stalled the placement of the warning on cigarette packages, "Smoking May Be Dangerous To Your Health," for five years, from 1964 to 1969. She lives in a two million dollar mansion in Georgetown, the former James Forrestal home.

The furor over lung cancer and smoking ignores a pertinent fact, that primitive tribes have been smoking tobacco for thousands of years, with no disagreeable after effects. In Virginia, origin of this writer, Indians were smoking tobacco when Captain John Smith landed at Jamestown. Dr. Richard Passey, a researcher at London's Chester Beattie Research Institute, conducted twenty years of research on the tobacco problem. He found no significant link between the traditionally air dried tobacco and lung cancer.

However, the American and English tobacco industries, which are dominated by the Rothschilds, use sugar in their tobacco, for a sweetened, sugar dried effect. England, uses 17% sugar, the United States 10%. England has the highest lung cancer rate in the world. Dr. Passey concluded that the addition of sugar to tobacco creates a carcinogenic substance in the nicotine tar; in air dried tobacco, this carcinogen is not activated. He found no resulting lung cancer in the Soviet Union, China and Taiwan, all of which produce air-dried tobacco.

Esquire magazine featured a lengthy article on the work of the Janker Clinic in Bonn, Germany, finding that this clinic has treated 76,000 cancer cases since 1936, with full or partial remission in 70% of their patients. The *Esquire* reporter was astounded to learn that "the National Cancer Institute refuses to use Janker Clinic isophosphamide, A. Mulsin, Wobe enzymes and other successful Janker techniques because they refused to use sufficient dosage. The American Cancer Society is even more rigid. It prides itself on keeping the Janker techniques out of the United States." The *Esquire* reporter went on to complain that "The American Cancer Society has become a major part of the problem. It eschews sponsorship of chemical and research innovation and instead goes in for propaganda (cigarettes are harmful, the Seven Danger Signals, celebrity radio and TV spots) and it virtually condemns and suppresses unorthodox methods which, incidentally, it does not even trouble itself to investigate thoroughly."

The reporter did not know that the American Cancer Society has a vested interest in the established forms of cancer treatment; for instance, it holds a fifty per cent ownership of the patent rights of 5 FU, (5 flourouracil), one the toxic drugs now in vogue as an "acceptable" medication for cancer. 5FU and a later development 5- 4-FU, are produced by Hoffman LaRoche Laboratories.

The Knight Ridder News Service reported in 1978 that the ACS refused to take a position on suspected pesticides which caused cancer. The ACS board and its allied organization, Sloan Kettering, have many members who are heads of the largest chemical firms in the United States. The war against pollution will win no adherents there. ACS was asked to take a position on other dangerous substances, such as Red Dye #2, the fire-retardant TRIS, used in children's clothing (it has since been banned), and forms of synthetic estrogen. Yet ACS again refused to state its position on these substances. To counter its baneful influence, the Committee for Freedom of Choice in Medicine planned to file an action in 1984 before the Permanent Committee on Human Rights at the United Nations, charging that the American medical establishment was in violation of the United Nations Declaration of Human Rights and the International Human Rights Agreement of 1966. Its prepared statement noted that "Americans have been needlessly slaughtered and criminalized because a host of useful products, medicine and metabolic nutritional approaches in medicine have been crushed by vested interests." The Committee termed the present situation "a Medigate."

The failure to reduce the death rate from cancer is a grim indictment of the insurmountable obstacles which the ACS has placed in the path of a viable approach to this problem. John Bailar of the Harvard School of Public Health, addressing the American Association for the Advancement of Science in 19867, pointed out that "The government's fifteen year old national cancer program has not lowered the death rate for major forms of cancer and should therefore be considered a failure. It has not produced the results it was supposed to produce." Bailar was well qualified to make this observation; he had been editor of the Journal for NCI for twenty- five years. He was supported by a fellow member of the faculty of the School of Public Health, Dr. John Cairns, who reported that, "In the past twenty years, cancer has increased; there have been no significant gains against cancer since the 1950s."

Dr. Hardin James addressed the ACS Panel in 1969. A professor of medical physics at the University of California at Berkely, he stated that his studies had proven conclusively that untreated cancer victims actually live up to four times longer than treated individuals. "For a typical type of cancer, people who refused treatment live an average of twelve and a half years. Those who accepted surgery and other kinds of treatment lived an average of only three years. I attribute this to the traumatic effect of surgery on the body's natural defense mechanism. The body has a natural type of defense against every type of cancer."

In February, 1988, the National Cancer Institute released its definitive report, summarizing the "war against cancer." It reported that over the past thirty-five years, both the overall incidence and death rates from cancer have increased, despite "advances" in detection and treatment." *Washington Post,* February 9, 1988. The problem may be that, just as in other wars we have engaged in the twentieth century, too many of those "on our side" are actually working for the enemy.

CHAPTER 4

VACCINATION

One of the few doctors who has dared to speak out against the Medical Monopoly, Dr. Robert S. Mendelsohn, dramatized his stand against Modern Medicine by defining it as a Church which has Four Holy Waters. The first of these, he listed as Vaccination. Dr. Mendelsohn termed vaccination "of questionable safety." However, other doctors have been more explicit. It is notable that the Rockefeller interests have fought throughout the nineteenth century to make these Four Holy Waters compulsory throughout the United States, ignoring all the protests and warnings of their dangers.

Of these four items, which might well be termed the Four Horsemen of the Apocalypse, because they too are known to bring death and destruction in their wake, the most pernicious in its longterm effects may well be the practice of immunization. This practice goes directly against the discovery of modern holistic medical experts that the body has a natural immune defense against illness. The Church of Modern Medicine claims that we can only be absolved from the peril of infection by the Holy Water of vaccination, injecting into the system a foreign body of infection, which will then perform a Medical Miracle, and will confer life-long immunity, hence the term, "immunization." The greatest heresy any physician can commit is to voice publicly any doubt of any one of the Four Holy Waters, but the most deeply entrenched in modern medical practice is undoubtedly the numerous vaccination programs. They are also the most consistently profitable operations of the Medical Monopoly. Yet one physician, Dr. Henry R. Bybee, of Norfolk, Virginia, has publicly stated, "My honest opinion is that vaccine is the cause of more disease and suffering than anything I could name. I believe that such diseases as cancer, syphilis, cold sores and many other disease conditions are the direct results of vaccination. Yet, in the state of Virginia, and in many other states, parents are compelled to submit their children to this procedure while the medical profession not only receives its pay for this service, but also makes splendid and prospective patients for the future."

The present writer well remembers the 1920s, as a child in Virginia, going to school for some weeks without having submitted to the compulsory vaccination ordered by the state authorities. Each morning, the teacher would begin the day's classes by asking, "Clarence, did you bring your vaccination certificate today?" Obviously, this was the most urgent business of the educational system, taking priority over such matters as lessons and studying. Each morning, I would have to reply, "No, I didn't bring it today." The other children would turn and stare at this dangerous classmate, who might infect them all with some terrible disease. My mother had been a registered nurse, and she never urged me to go ahead with my vaccination. I suspect she knew more than the doctors about its possible effects. After postponing the dreaded ordeal for some weeks, I was finally led to the doctor like an animal being led up the plank to be stunned, and I received my injection. Of course it made me extremely ill, as my body fought the infection, but the class was delivered from peril, and I was accepted as a duly branded member of society. In "The Curse of Canaan," I wrote of the deliverance of our children up for ritual sacrifice, a practice which seemingly ended with the destruction of the Baal cult some five thousand years ago. Unfortunately, the Cult of Baal seems to be firmly entrenched in the present

Establishment, which is often known by the sobriquet, the Brotherhood of Death. It is disturbing to see how the educationists eagerly embrace each new offense against children in our schools, railing against any mention of morality or religion, while solemnly indoctrinating six year olds in the advantages of "an alternative life style" in their sexual preferences. The present goal of the National Education Association seems to be that teachers should hand out condoms to the class before beginning each day's activities.

The urgency of my vaccination was not that there was any epidemic then raging in the city of Roanoke, nor has there been one in the ensuing sixty years. The urgency was that no child shall be spared the ministrations of the Cult of Baal, or forego sacrifice on the altar of the child molesters. The Medical Monopoly cannot afford to have a single pupil escape the monetary offering to be paid for the compulsory vaccination, the tribute of the enslaved to their masters.

From London comes an alarming observation from a practitioner of excellent reputation and long experience. Dr. Herbert Snow, senior surgeon at the Cancer Hospital of London, voiced his concern, "In recent years many men and women in the prime of life have dropped dead suddenly, often after attending a feast or a banquet. I am convinced that some eighty per cent of these deaths are caused by the inoculation or vaccination they have undergone. They are well known to cause grave and permanent disease to the heart. The coroner always hushes it up as 'natural causes.' "

You cannot find any such warning in any medical textbook or popular book on health. In fact, this writer was able to locate it in a small volume buried deep in the stacks of the Library of Congress. Yet such an ominous observation from an established medical practitioner should be as widely circulated as possible, if only to be attached by those who can refute its premise. At least it cannot be attacked by the Establishment as quackery, because Dr. Snow is not attempting to sell some substitute for vaccination, but merely warning of its dangers.

Another practitioner, Dr. W. B. Clarke of Indiana, finds that "Cancer was practically unknown until compulsory vaccination with cowpox vaccine began to be introduced. I have had to deal with a least two hundred cases of cancer, and I never saw a case of cancer in an unvaccinated person."

At last, we have the breakthrough for which the American Cancer Society has been searching, at such great expense, and for so many years. Dr. Clarke has never seen a case of cancer in an unvaccinated person. Is not this a lead which should be explored?

With such an impetus, the ACS could once again get the telephone banks ringing in the fund-raising drives, to initiate positive research as to the possible connection between vaccination and the incidence of cancer. Somehow, we suspect that ACS will not follow this lead. It would also look well etched in stone above the imposing entrance to the Memorial Sloan Kettering Cancer Center, "I never saw a case of cancer in an unvaccinated person." However, it is unlikely that the High Priests of Modern Medicine will be able to give up one of the Four Commandments. It will be necessary for an outraged public to bring pressure to bear to abandon the modern ritual of sacrificing our children to Baal in a five thousand year old ritual called, in its modern version, "compulsory immunization."

In the land where freedom rings, or is supposed to ring, it is even more surprising to find that every citizen is compelled to submit to a compulsory vaccination ritual. Here again, we are speaking of a civilization which is now being visited by two plagues, the plague of cancer and the plague of AIDS, yet compulsory vaccination offers no protection against the plagues which threaten us. It is goodbye whooping cough, goodbye diptheria and hello AIDS. The Medical Monopoly is searching desperately for some type of "immunization" against these plagues, and no doubt will eventually come up with some type of "vaccine" which will be more dreadful than the disease. From the outset, our most distinguished medical experts have proudly informed us that AIDS is incurable, which is hardly the approach we expect from those who demand that we accept their infallibility in all things to do with medicine.

Another wellknown medical practitioner, Dr. J. M. Peebles of San Francisco, has written a book on vaccine, in which he says, "The vaccination practice, pushed to the front on all occasions by the medical profession through political connivance made compulsory by the state, has not only become the chief menace and the greatest danger to the health of the rising generation, but likewise the crowning outrage upon the personal liberties of the American citizen; compulsory vaccination, poisoning the crimson currents of the human system with brute-extracted lymph under the strange infatuation that it would prevent smallpox, was one of the darkest blots that disfigured the last century."

Dr. Peebles refers to the fact that cowpox vaccine was one of the more peculiar "inventions or discoveries of the Age of Enlightenment." However, as I have pointed out in "*The Curse of Canaan*,"[1] the Age of Enlightenment was merely the latest program of the Cult of Baal and its rituals of child sacrifice, which, in one guise or another, has now been with us for some five thousand years. Because of this goal, the

---

[1] Published by Omnia Veritas Ltd.

Medical Monopoly is also known as "The Society for Crippling Children."

Perhaps the most telling comment of Dr. Peebles' criticism is his reference to "brute-extracted lymph." Could there be some connection between the injection of this substance and the spread of a hitherto unknown form of cancer, cancer of the lymph glands?

This type of cancer is not only one of the most commonly encountered versions of this disease; it is also one of the most difficult to treat, because it rapidly spreads throughout the entire system. A diagnosis of cancer of the lymph glands now means a virtual death sentence.

If we suppose that physicians such as Dr. Snow and Dr. Peebles are trumpeting nonexistent dangers when they write of vaccination, we have only to look at the court records of many cases around the country. Wyeth Laboratories was the defendant in a case in which a Wichita Kansas jury recently awarded $15 million in damages to an eight year old girl. She incurred permanent brain damage after receiving a diptheria-pertussis-tetanus vaccine. Michelle Graham received the immunization at the age of three months, and incurred severe brain damage which left her permanently incapacitated. Her lawyers proved that the damage was solely attributable to the vaccine, although Wyeth's lawyers attempted to deny this.

Because of the financial prospects, physicians are demanding earlier vaccination for children each year. The Vaccination Committee of the American Academy of Pediatricians recently demanded that the age for children to receive flu vaccine be lowered from the previous twenty-four months to eighteen months. They are promoting a new version of flu vaccine which was said to have been tested on children in Finland.

In an article in *Science,* March 4, 1977, Jonas and Darrell Salk warn that, "Live virus vaccines against influenza or poliomyelitis may in each instance produce the disease it intended to prevent ... the live virus against measles and mumps may produce such side effects as encephalitis (brain damage)."

If vaccines present such a clear and present danger to children who are forced to submit to them, we must examine the forces which demand that they submit. In the United States, vaccines are actively and incessantly promoted as the solution for all infectious diseases by such government agencies as the Center for Disease Control in Georgia, by HEW, USPHS, FDA, AMA and WHO. It is of more than passing interest that the federal agencies should be such passionate supporters of compulsory use of vaccines, and that they also should go through the "revolving door" to the big drug firms whose products they have so assiduously promoted, throughout their years of service to the public. It is these federal agents who have drafted the procedures which forced the states to enact compulsory vaccination legislation which had been drafted by the attorneys for the Medical Monopoly, to become "the law of the land." In the dim reaches of the past, when Americans were more protective of their now-vanishing freedoms, there was sporadic opposition to the threatened outrage which a dictatorial central government sought to impose on every child in the United States. In 1909, the Senate of the Commonwealth of Massachusetts introduced Bill No. 8; "An Act To Prohibit Compulsory Vaccine. Sec. 1. It shall be unlawful for any board of education, board of health, or any public board acting in this state, under political regulations or otherwise, to compel by resolution, order or proceedings of any kind, the vaccination of any child or person of any age, by making vaccination a condition precedent to the attending of any public or private school, either as pupil or teacher."

No doubt this legislation was drafted by a physician who was well aware of the dangers of vaccination. Even in 1909, the Medical Monopoly was strong enough to bury this bill. It was never submitted for vote. However, the peril of even one state legislature foiling their criminal conspiracy caused the Rockefeller Syndicate to concentrate on perfecting an instrument for controlling each and every state legislature in these United States. This was achieved by setting up the Council of State Governments in Chicago. Its ukases are routinely issued to every state legislator, and such is its totalitarian control that not one legislature has ever failed to follow its dictates.

Edward Jenner (1796-1839) "discovered" that cowpox vaccine would supposedly inoculate persons against the eighteenth century scourge of smallpox. In fact, smallpox was already on the wane, and some authorities believe it would have vanished by the end of the century, due to a number of contributing factors. After the use of cowpox vaccine became widespread in England, a smallpox epidemic broke out which killed 22,081 people. The smallpox epidemics became worse each year that the vaccine was used. In 1872, 44,480 people were killed by it. England finally banned the vaccine in 1948, despite the fact that it was one of the most widely heralded "contributions" which that country had made to modern medicine. This action came after many years of compulsory vaccination, during which period those who refused to submit to its dangers were hurried off to jail.

Japan initiated compulsory vaccine in 1872. In 1892, there were 165,774 cases of smallpox there, which resulted in 29,979 deaths.

Japan still enforces compulsory vaccination; however, since it is a militarily occupied nation, its present government can hardly be blamed for submitting to the Rockefeller Medical Monopoly.

Germany also instituted compulsory vaccination. In 1939 (this during the Nazi regime), the diptheria rate increased astronomically to 150,000 cases. Norway, which never instituted compulsory vaccination, had only fifty cases during the same period. Polio has increased 700% in states which have compulsory vaccination. The much quoted writer on medical problems, Morris Beale, who for years edited his informative publication, *Capsule News Digest, from Capitol Hill*, offered a standing reward during the years from 1954 to 1960 of $30,000, which he would pay to anyone who could prove that the polio vaccine was not a killer and a fraud. There were no takers.

Medical historians have finally come to the reluctant conclusion that the great flu "epidemic" of 1918 was solely attributable to the widespread use of vaccines. It was the first war in which vaccination was compulsory for all servicemen. The *Boston Herald* reported that forty-seven soldiers had been killed by vaccination in one month. As a result, the military hospitals were filled, not with wounded combat casualties, but with casualties of the vaccine. The epidemic was called "the Spanish Influenza," a deliberately misleading appellation, which was intended to conceal its origin. This flu epidemic claimed twenty million victims; those who survived it were the ones who had refused the vaccine. In recent years, annual recurring epidemics of flu are called "the Russian Flu." For some reason, the Russians never protest, perhaps because the Rockefellers make regular trips to Moscow to lay down the party line.

The perils of vaccination were already known. *Plain Talk* magazine notes that "during the Franco-Prussian War, every German soldier was vaccinated. The result was that 53,288 otherwise healthy men developed smallpox. The death rate was high."

In what is now known as "the Great Swine Flu Massacre," the President of the United States, Gerald Ford, was enlisted to persuade the public to undergo a national vaccination campaign. The moving force behind the scheme was a $135 million windfall profit for the major drug manufacturers. They had a "swine flu" vaccine which suspicious pig raisers had refused to touch, fearful it might wipe out their crop. The manufacturers had only tried to get $80 million from the swine breeders; balked in this sale, they turned to the other market, humans. The impetus for the national swine flu vaccine came directly from the Disease Control Center in Atlanta, Georgia. Perhaps coincidentally, Jimmy Carter, a member of the Trilateral Commission, was then planning his presidential campaign in Georgia. The incumbent President, Gerald Ford, had all the advantages of a massive bureaucracy to aid him in his election campaign, while the ineffectual and little known Jimmy Carter offered no serious threat in the election. Suddenly, out of Atlanta, came the Center of Disease Control plan for a national immunization campaign against "swine flu." The fact that there was not a single known case of this flu in the United States did not deter the Medical Monopoly from their scheme. The swine breeders had been shocked by the demonstrations of the vaccine on a few pigs, which had collapsed and died. One can imagine the anxious conferences in the headquarters of the great drug firms, until one bright young man remarked, "Well, if the swine breeders won't inject it into their animals, our only other market is to inject it into people."

The Ford sponsored swine flu campaign almost died an early death, when a conscientious public servant, Dr. Anthony Morris, formerly of HEW and then active as director of the Virus Bureau at the Food and Drug

Administration, declared that there could be no authentic swine flu vaccine, because there had never been any cases of swine flu on which they could test it. Dr. Morris then went public with his statement that "at no point were the swine flu vaccines effective." He was promptly fired, but the damage had been done.

The damage control consisted of that great humanitarian, Walter Cronkite, and the President of the United States, combining their forces to come to the rescue of the Medical Monopoly. Walter Cronkite had President Ford appear on his news program to urge the American people to submit to the inoculation with the swine flu vaccine. CBS then or later could never find any reason to air any analysis or scientific critique of the swine flu vaccine, which was identified as containing many toxic poisons, including alien viral protein particles, formaldehyde, residues of chicken and egg embryo substances, sucrose, theimorosal (a derivative of poisonous mercury), polysorbate and some eighty other substances.

Meanwhile, back at the virus laboratories, after Dr. Anthony Morris has been summarily fired, a special team of workers was rushed in to clean out the four rooms in which he had conducted his scientific tests. The laboratory was filled with animals whose records verified his claims, representing some three years of constant research. All of the animals were immediately destroyed, and Morris' records were burned. They did not go so far as to sow salt throughout the area, because they believed their job was done.

On April 15, 1976, Congress passed Public Law 94-266, which provided $135 million of taxpayers' funds to pay for a national swine flu inoculation campaign. HEW was to distribute the vaccine to state and local health agencies on a national basis for inoculation, at no charge. Insurance agencies then went public with their warning that they would not insure drug firms against possible suits from the results of swine flu inoculation, because no studies had been carried out which could predict its effects. It was to foil the insurance companies that CBS had Gerald Ford make his impassioned appeal to 215,000,000 Americans to save themselves while there was still time, and to rush down to the friendly local health department and get the swine flu vaccination, at absolutely no charge. This may have been CBS' finest hour in its distinguished career of "public service."

Hardly had the swine flu campaign been completed than the reports of the casualties began to pour in. Within a few months, claims totalling $1.3 billion had been filed by victims who had suffered paralysis from the swine flu vaccine. The medical authorities proved equal to the challenge; they leaped to the defense of the Medical Monopoly by labeling the new epidemic, "Guillain- Barre Syndrome." There have since been increasing speculations that the ensuing epidemic of AIDS which began shortly after Gerald Ford's public assurances, was merely a viral variation of the swine flu vaccine. And what of the perpetrator of the Great Swine Flu Massacre, President Gerald Ford? As the logical person to blame for the catastrophe, Ford had to endure a torrent of public criticism, which quite naturally resulted in his defeat for election (he had previously been appointed when the agents of the international drug operations had ushered Richard Nixon out of office). The unknown Jimmy Carter, familiar only to the supersecret fellow members in the Trilateral Commission, was swept into office by the outpouring of rage against Gerald Ford. Carter proved to be almost as serious a national disaster as the swine flu epidemic, while Gerald Ford was retired from politics to life. Not only did he lose the election; he was also sentenced to spend his remaining years trudging wearily up and down the hot sandy stretches of the Palm Springs Golf course.

At the annual ACS Science Writers Seminar, Dr. Robert W. Simpson, of Rutgers University, warned that "immunization programs against flu, measles, mumps and polio may actually be seeding humans with RNA to form proviruses which will then become latent cells throughout the body. they can then become activated as a variety of diseases including lupus, cancer, rheumatism and arthritis."

This was a remarkable verification of the earlier warning delivered by Dr. Herbert Snow of London more than fifty years earlier. He had observed that the long-term effects of the vaccine, lodging in the heart or other parts of the body, would eventually result in fatal damage to the heart. The vaccine becomes a time bomb in the system, festering as what are known as "slow viruses," which may take ten to thirty years to become virulent. When that time arrives, the victim is felled by a fatal onslaught, often with no prior warning, whether it is a heart attack or some other disease.

Health Freedom News, in its July/August 1986 issue, noted that "Vaccine is linked to brain damage. 150 lawsuits pending against DPT vaccine manufacturers, seeking $1.5 billion damages."

When the present writer was a teenager in Virginia, each summer became a nightmare for anxious parents, as epidemics of poliomyelitis, generally called infantile paralysis, swept the nation. Throughout the summer, we imbibed bottle after bottle of ice cold soda pop to wash down our afternoon snacks of candy bars, with no inkling that we were preparing our systems for the breeding of the polio virus. The most famous victim of polio was the Governor of New York, Franklin D. Roosevelt. In 1931, during the annual polio epidemic, Roosevelt officially endorsed a so-called "immune serum," a precursor of the polio vaccines of the 1950s. It was sponsored by Dr. Lindsly R. Williams, the son-in-law of the managing partner of the investment bankers,

Kidder Peabody. The Rockefeller and Carnegie Foundations had urged the building of a new medical edifice to be called the New York Academy of Medicine. As was often the case, they did not provide the funds, but planned the staging campaign whereby the public was induced to contribute millions of dollars for it. Dr. Williams was then appointed director of this Academy, despite the fact that his medical abilities were a joke in New York. Williams used this post to become the apostle of socialized medicine in the United States, a goal which the Rockefeller Medical Monopoly ardently desired, and which was finally achieved when the Medicare program was adopted many years later. In reality, as Dr. Emanuel Josephson pointed out, Williams stood for the political and commercial domination of the medical profession under a socialized system.

Roosevelt then announced his candidacy for the Presidency of the United States, a post for which he seemed physically disqualified. Because of his handicap, he had been unable to stand or walk for many years. He conducted his business from a wheelchair. It seemed incredible that he would be able to wage a national campaign for the office of president. To allay these doubts, Dr. Williams wrote an article which was published in *Collier's* magazine, the second largest magazine in the United States at that time. In this article, Dr. Williams certified that Governor Franklin D. Roosevelt was physically and mentally fit to be President of the United States. It was then bruited about that a new Cabinet post, Secretary of Health, was to be created especially for Dr. Williams in an upcoming Roosevelt Administration.

The "immune serum" against polio was known to be dangerous and worthless when Roosevelt endorsed it. The National Health Institute of the U.S. Public Health Service had experimented with monkeys for three years, using this identical serum. The Institute stated that a study of the serum had been made on the recommendation of Dr. Simon Flexner, the head of the Institute. The serum was then used, and many children died from it. The New York State Commissioner of Health, Dr. Thomas Parran (who was later appointed Surgeon General of the United States), who owed his appointment to Dr. Williams' recommendation to Governor Roosevelt, refused to hold hearings to validate the serum, while Roosevelt continued to reap the rewards of "charity" from his Warm Springs Foundation and his annual birthday balls celebrating the polio epidemic.

In 1948, a Dr. Sandler, who was then serving as nutritional expert at the U.S. Veterans Administration Hospital in Oteen, North Carolina, became alarmed at the enormous amounts of heavily sugared drinks, candy and other sweets which were being consumed by children during the hot summer months, at the same time that the polio became epidemic each year. He conducted tests which led him to the conclusion that the children's consumption of sugar had a direct relation to the virulence of the polio outbreaks. He then issued an urgent warning to parents to ban consumption of any refined sugar product, particularly candy, soft drinks and ice cream during the summer months. The result of Dr. Sandler's campaign was that the number of polio cases dropped in North Carolina 90% in a single year, from 2,498 in 1948 to only 229 in 1949. Aroused by the effect that Dr. Sandler's warning campaign had had on their summer sales in North Carolina, the soft drink distributors and the candy manufacturers came in the following year with a statewide promotional campaign, featuring free samples and other promotions. By 1950, the polio toll had risen once more to its 1948 level. What happened to Dr. Sandler? A study of North Carolina publications shows no further mention of him or his program.

Herbert M. Shelton wrote in 1938 in his book, "Exploitation of Human Suffering," that "Vaccine is pus—

either septic or inert—if inert it will not take—if septic it produces infection." This explains why some children have to go back and receive a second inoculation, because the first one did not "take"—it was not sufficiently poisonous, and did not infect the body. Shelton says that the inoculations cause sleeping sickness, infantile paralysis, haemoplagia or tetanus.

The Surgeon General of the United States, Leonard Scheele, pointed out to the annual AMA convention in 1955 that "No batch of vaccine can be proven safe before it is given to children." James R. Shannon of the National Institute of Health declared that "The only safe vaccine is a vaccine that is never used."

With the advent of Dr. Jonas Salk's polio vaccine in the 1950s American parents were assured that the problem had been solved, and that their children were now safe. The ensuing suits against the drug manufacturers received little publicity. "David v. Wyeth Labs," a suit involving Type 3 Sabin Polio Vaccine, was judged in favor of the plaintiff, David. A suit against Lederle Lab involving Orimune Vaccine was settled in 1962 for $10,000. In two cases involving Parke-Davis' Quadrigen, the product was found to be defective. In 1962, Parke-Davis halted all production of Quadrigen. The medical loner, Dr. William Koch, declared that "The injection of any serum, vaccine, or even penicillin has shown a very marked increase in the incidence of polio, at least by 400%."

The Center for Disease Control stayed out of sight for some time after the Great Swine Flu Massacre, only to emerge more stridently than ever with a new national scare program on the dangers of another plague, which was named "Legionnaires' Disease" after an outbreak at the Bellevue Stratford Hotel in Philadelphia. Apparently this virus multiplied in the air conditioning and heating systems of some older hotels in large cities, probably because the vents were never cleaned. In a few isolated instances, it caused death to those who were afflicted. For some reason, these victims were usually elderly Legionnaires, who had attended a gathering at one of these hotels. As the older hotels were gradually replaced by new, more modern motels, Legionnaires Disease quietly faded away, without the Disease Control Center being able to bring off another $135 million coup for the Rockefeller Medical Monopoly.

Polio vaccination has now been accepted as a fact of life by the American public, which derives considerable comfort from the gradual disappearance of the annual scare campaign at the beginning of each summer. . . However, the *Washington Post* of January 26, 1988 featured a story which created some puzzling afterthoughts. It was announced at a national conference held in Washington that all

cases of polio since 1979 had been caused by the polio vaccine. We quote, "In fact, all the cases in America come from the vaccine. The naturally occurring (or wild type) polio virus has not been shown to cause a single case of polio in the United States since 1979." It was to confront this unpleasant fact that the Institute of Medicine, under contract to the U.S. Public Health Service, had convened a committee in Washington to review the current use of polio vaccine. You thought they would vote to discontinue it, perhaps? This would be a logical conclusion. Unfortunately, logic plays no part in such deliberations. The *Post* reported that "No radical change is expected. 'The status quo is very appealing,' " said conference chairman Dr. Frederick Robbins, of Case Western Reserve University in Cleveland.

This story raises more questions than it answers. It also reveals the wide gap between the medical mind and that of the layman. A layman would say, "If all cases of polio in the United States since 1979 have been caused by the polio vaccine, isn't this a good reason for discontinuing?" Such reasoning is always called "simplistic" by our overeducated professionals. After all, one has to think of the national economy, and of drug manufacturers geared up to the continuous production of a vaccine for an epidemic which has disappeared. Think of the unemployment, and the diminution of dividends to the holders of stock in the Drug Trust. After all, most of their income is donated to "charity." If you cannot see the logic of this reasoning, you will never get a job with the U.S. Public Health Service.

CHAPTER 5

FLUORIDATION

The second item on Dr. Robert Mendelsohn's list of the Four Holy Waters of the modern Church of Medicine is the fluoridation of the nation's drinking water. Although Dr. Mendelsohn dismisses it too, as of "questionable value," few dare to question it. We are told that it confers untold benefits to the rising generation, guaranteeing them perpetual freedom from tooth decay and no need for any dental work. Surprisingly enough, the national fluoridation campaign is enthusiastically supported by the nation's dental profession, even though it might be expected that it would put them out of business. Here again, those in the know are well aware that the fluoridation program, far from threatening to put the dentists out of business, actually will offer them plenty of work in the future.

The principal source of the fluoridation is a poisonous chemical, sodium fluoride, which has long been the principal ingredient of rat poison. Whether the adding of this compound to our drinking water is also part of a rat control program has never been publicly discussed. The EPA released its latest estimate, that 38 million Americans are now drinking unsafe water, which contains unsafe levels of chlorine, lead and other toxic substances. Fluoride is not listed as one of the toxic substances. EPA, like other government agencies, has carefully refrained from either testing public drinking water for the effects of fluoridation, or from poaching on the preserves of the Rockefeller

Monopoly, which launched the national fluoridation campaign.

The by-product of the manufacture of aluminum, sodium fluoride, had long posed a problem. Except for its limited use as a rat poison, other popular uses were limited by its extremely poisonous nature. It also was very expensive for the aluminum companies to dispose of, because of its persistence (it does not degrade—it is also cumulative in the body, so that each day you add a little more to your sodium fluoride reserves each time you drink a glass of water). It is puzzling, then, to find that the historical record shows that the principal sponsor and promoter of the fluoridation of the nation's drinking water was the U.S. Public Health Service. And thereby hangs a tale.

We may recall the heady days of the 1950s, when public health officials were routinely sent out from Washington to appear at meetings where communities were anxiously debating the pros and cons of water fluoridation. Without exception, these public servants not only reassured the anxious citizens, they positively demanded that the communities fluoridate then-drinking water. Although they unequivocally endorsed the fluoridation of water supplies, not one of these public health officials had ever conducted any studies of fluoridated water, or made any experiments as to its possible benefits or dangers. Yet at meeting after meeting throughout the United States, they rose to solemnly guarantee that there were no dangers, no side effects, only positive benefits on children under the age of twelve. Fluoridation, even according to its most enthusiastic supporters, confers no benefits on anyone older than twelve. No sensible reason has ever been advanced as to why all water supplies should be fluoridated, in order to benefit a minority of the population. Did these public servants know what they were doing? Of course not. They were following a tradition of the bureaucracy, which takes its orders from the

Medical Monopoly. How did they get these orders? That too, is an interesting story.[2]

The head of the U.S. Public Health Service during the entire fluoridation campaign was one Oscar Ewing. A graduate of Harvard Law School, Ewing was an airplane contractor during the First World War. He then joined the influential law firm of Sherman, Hughes and Dwight, a prestigious Wall Street Company. The "Hughes" was none other than Charles Evans Hughes, the recent candidate for the Presidency of the United States. Hughes lost his campaign against Woodrow Wilson because Wilson campaigned on his record, that "He kept us out of the war." As soon as he was safely re-elected, Wilson declared war. Hughes later became Chief Justice of the Supreme Court. The firm was then Ewing and Hughes.

At the end of World War II, Ewing had himself appointed a Special Prosecutor for the Department of Justice; the appointment was made solely to conduct two prosecutions for the Rockefeller Monopoly, the government's cases against two radio broadcasters, William Dudley Pelley and Robert Best. Both of these writers, longtime activists in America First, had campaigned to keep the United States out of what had turned out to be a very profitable war. They now had to be punished for their threat to the monopolists.

---

[2] The U.S. Public Health Service continues to propagandize (at taxpayers' expense) for expansion of fluoridation. The Washington Post noted on April 20, 1988 that "The Public Health Service estimates that each year $2 billion is saved through water fluoridation." Our Public Health Service demurs on any statistical substantiation for this claim. Do the Public Health Service officials imply that the aluminum manufacturers save $2 billion a year through fluoridation of water?

Ewing had them both convicted and sent to prison. For this service, he was then appointed chairman of the Democratic National Committee. The following year, in 1946, President Truman appointed him head of the Federal Security Agency. In this capacity, he was in nominal charge of another radio broadcaster, Ezra Pound, who was being held as a political prisoner at St. Elizabeths Hospital, a federal mental institution which was also part of the Federal Security Agency's network. Pound was held for more than thirteen years without trial. Long after Ewing had gone, the government dropped all charges against Pound, and he was freed.

However, Ewing had not been appointed Administrator of the Federal Security Agency merely to prosecute Ezra Pound. There were more serious goals in view. Congressman Miller charged that Ewing had been paid a $750,000 fee to leave his profitable Wall Street practice and head the Federal Security Agency. This fee had been paid by the Rockefeller interests. The purpose was to pursue a national fluoridation campaign. Ewing was made head of the Federal Security Agency because this position made him the most powerful bureaucrat in Washington. This agency encompassed the

U.S. Public Health Service, the Social Security Administration, and the Office of Education. As head of the FSA, he was in charge of the vast government postwar spending programs, the federal health, education and welfare programs. From this post, Ewing campaigned for greater government control over the citizens of the United States. He was particularly anxious to increase control of medical education, a prime goal of the Rockefeller interests since 1898. On February 17, 1948, Ewing publicly called for government grants for medical scholarships, and demanded that medical schools be operated under government subsidies, with the inevitable accompanying control. On

March 30, 1948, Ewing chaired a Children's Conference, which was intended to coordinate all federal agencies which had any dealing with the nation's youth. He also became the national leader of a campaign against cancer, a result of his long association with the Drug Trust—he had been secretary of the giant Merck Drug Company from his offices at One Wall Street.

One of Ewing's first moves as head of the Public Health Service was to throw out the longtime Surgeon General, Thomas Parran, replacing him with an Ewing crony, Dr. Leonard Scheele from the National Cancer Institute. In 1948, Ewing joined with the American Cancer Society in a National Campaign Against Cancer, a flagrant attempt to force Congress to spend more on various cancer boondoggles than the then modest expenditure of fourteen and a half million dollars a year. On May 1, 1948, Ewing convened a National Health Convention in Washington, with some 800 delegates in attendance. The convention overwhelmingly approved Ewing's plea to enroll the United States in the United Nations' World Health Organization. Ewing also campaigned vigorously for national health insurance, or socialized medicine, but despite his great power in Washington, he was unable to overcome the continued opposition of Morris Fishbein and the American Medical Association. He then issued an official report from the Federal Security Agency, "The Nation's Health," a 186 page report which called for a crash ten year program to achieve his goal of socialized medicine in the United States. The climax of his political power came when he masterminded Harry Truman's successful campaign for election to the Presidency in 1948 (Truman had previously succeeded as heir apparent after the strange death of Franklin D. Roosevelt (see Dr. Emanuel Josephson's book with that title). Ewing had already singlehandedly obtained the naming of Truman as the vice presidential campaign in the 1944 Chicago Convention—he could be said to have put

Truman in the White House as certainly as Bobst was later to put in Richard Nixon. The 1948 election of Truman guaranteed Ewing that he could have anything he wanted in Washington. What he wanted, and what he had been paid to bring about, was the national fluoridation of our drinking water.

Oscar Ewing is a name totally unknown to Americans today.

He left no monuments, because he was the twentieth century epitome of the ruthless, dedicated Soviet style of bureaucrat, answerable only to his masters, and contemptuous of the faceless masses over whom he exercised dictatorial powers. He wielded absolute control over the most important components of the new socialist bureaucracy which Roosevelt had built up in Washington, and he prepared these offices for Cabinet status. Of his many bureaucratic mandates, perhaps none has had a more direct effect on all Americans than the fluoridation of our water supply.

Congressman Miller stated that "The chief supporter of the fluoridation of water is the U.S. Public Health Service. This is part of Mr. Ewing's Federal Security Agency. Mr. Ewing is one of the highly paid lawyers for the Aluminum Company of America." It was hardly accidental that Washington, D.C., where Oscar Ewing was king, was one of the first large American cities to fluoridate its water supply. At the same time, Congressmen and other politicians in Washington were privately alerted by Ewing's minions that they should be careful about ingesting the fluoridated water. Supplies of bottled water from mountain springs then appeared in every office on Capitol Hill; these have been maintained continuously ever since, at the taxpayers' expense. One Senator, who went so far as to carry a small flask of spring water with him when he dined at

Washington's most fashionable restaurants, assuring his dinner companions that "Not one drop of fluoridated water will ever pass my lips." Such are the guardians of our nation.

Even without such government additives as chlorine and fluorine, water itself may pose a serious threat to health. American pioneers often came down with an illness which they called "milk sickness," which seems to have come from their water. Dr. N. M. Walker warns that in the average seventy year life span, the system ingests about 4,500 gallons of water containing some 300 pounds of lime. This intake of lime gradually ossifies the skeletal structure. In 1845, an English physician warned of the peril of ossification from drinking natural or spring water.

When Congressman Miller reported on the floor of Congress that Oscar Ewing was promoting fluoridation because he had been the lawyer for the Aluminum Company of America, ALCOA, and that he had accepted a $750,000 "fee" to persuade him to undertake this program of "government service," one would have thought that this public exposure of Ewing's motives would have shamed him, and perhaps influence him to step aside and let someone else take over the U.S. Public Health Service campaign to force fluoridation on the American people. This would underestimate the arrogance and the self-assurance of the twentieth century bureaucrat. He ignored Congressman's Miller's remarks, and redoubled the pressure of the U.S. Public Health Service to put over fluoridation. He had the willing support of his underlings, because the U.S. Public Health Service has never been in the service of the public. On the contrary, its officials have always been at the beck and call of the Drug Trust, pushing the latest fads from the Medical Monopoly, and maintaining those ideals of public service which have purchased so many fine estates in the fashionable Leesburg suburban area for those who have been in the right place at the right time. Political power is translated into money; money for those who use political goals for sale.

After overseeing the installation of sodium fluoride equipment in most of the nation's large cities, an interest in which Chase Manhattan Bank showed a crucial concern, Oscar Ewing retired to Chapel Hill, N.C. in 1953. Here he busied himself with building a 7,800 acre complex of office buildings under the name of the Research Triangle Corporation (triangle being a key Masonic symbol). These offices were promptly leased to a melange of federal and state agencies, many of which, not surprisingly, he had previously done business with when he was their boss in Washington. A former head of the Democratic National Committee usually has no difficulty in renting space to government agencies.

Ewing's former law partner, Charles Evans Hughes, Jr., became Solicitor General of the United States, while his father was still Chief Justice of the Supreme Court. He later became a director of New York Life Insurance Co., a J. P. Morgan controlled firm, whose office was at One Wall Street. This had also been Oscar Ewing's former business address.

Fluorides have long been a source of contamination in the United States. Large quantities of this chemical are also produced by the giant chemical firms, American Agricultural Products Corporation, and Hooker Chemical. Hooker Chemical became part of the Rockefeller network when Blanchette Hooker married into the Rockefeller family by marrying John D. Rockefeller III. The Florida plant of American Agricultural produces enormous waste quantities of fluorides in preparing fertilizer from phosphate rock.

Some of the fluoride wastes had been used in pesticides, until the Department of Agriculture banned their use as being too dangerous to the public. The wastes were then dumped into the ocean, despite specific Department of Agriculture rulings prohibiting it. Hooker Chemical is known to most Americans for the life-threatening chemical wastes found at Love Canal.

Studies by the National Academy of Science show that United States industries such as Hooker Chemical pump 100,000 tons of fluorides into the atmosphere each year; they pipe another 500,000 tons of fluorides into the nations water supply each year (this is in addition to the amount of fluorides used in "treating" our drinking water). This scientific report further analyzes the effects of these fluorides on the human system. Its most dangerous effect is that it slows down the vitally important DNA repair enzyme activity of the immune system. Fluorides have this effect even in concentrations as low as one part per million, the standard dosage which the U.S. Public Health Service set for our drinking water. At this concentration, fluorides are shown to cause serious chromosomal damage. The one part per million recommended by our conscientious public servants has also been shown in laboratory experiments to transform normal cells into cancer cells. American Academy of Science studies in 1963 showed that these "low" levels of fluorides resulted in a marked increase in melanotic tumors, from 12% to 100% in experimental laboratory animals. It also caused interference with the body's production of important neurotransmitters, and lowered their level in the brain. These neurotransmitters have the vital function of protecting against seizures, thus opening the possibility of major increases in strokes and brain damage because of the fluorides in water. Lesser effects of fluorides which have been noted in laboratory tests are sudden mood changes, severe headaches, nausea, hallucinations, irregular breathing, night twitching, damage to fetuses, and various forms of cancer.

Government objections to these laboratory findings were raised by the quintessential bureaucrat, Dr. Frank J. Rauscher, the director of the National Cancer Institute, when he claimed that "Scientists within and without the National Cancer Program have found again that the fluoridation of drinking water does not contribute to a cancer burden for people." This claim, for which he offered no scientific verification, was sharply contested by a longtime scholar of the fluoridation controversy, Dr. John Yiamouyiannis, Dean Burk and other scientists. In his authoritative work, "Fluoride: The Aging Factor," which has never been refuted by any scientific study, Dr. Yiamouyiannis finds that from thirty thousand to fifty thousand deaths a year are directly traceable to fluoridation, from ten to twenty thousand of these deaths being from fluoride induced cancers.

Although some communities have since revoked their agreements to allow fluoridation of their public drinking water supplies, the national campaign continues unabated. No government official has ever admitted that there might be dangers associated with the Ewing bribe which resulted in the fluoridation of the nation's drinking water. West Germany banned fluoridation November 18, 1971, which was surprising because this is a militarily occupied nation, which is run by the top secret German Marshall Fund and the John J. McCloy Foundation. Apparently they could no longer silence the German scientists who have proved that fluoridation is a deadly threat to the population. Sweden followed West Germany in banning fluoridation, and the Netherlands officially banned it on June 22, 1973, by order of their highest court.

It is of some interest to contemplate the process by which the government bureaucrats arrived at the recommended dosage for fluoridating public drinking water, that is, one part per million.

Extensive studies must have been made, deliberations gone over by distinguished scientists over a period of years, before it was finally determined that this was the correct dosage. In fact, no such studies were ever made. Apparently the figure of one part per million was selected arbitrarily. It was known that ten parts per million was much too strong; after several years of using the one part per million dosage, government bureaucrats realized that they had made a terrible mistake. The dosage was at least twice as strong as it should have been. The death rates among elderly people from kidney and heart disease began to rise steadily in the first cities to begin fluoridating their water. One critic believes this was a deliberate decision, the "final solution" to the problem of Social Security payments. When scientists found that one part per million dosage of fluoridation transforms normal cells into cancerous cells, the fluoridation program should have been halted immediately. The government agencies realized that if they did so, they would open the door for thousands of lawsuits against the government.

Therefore, the stealthy poisoning of our older generation continues. Oscar Ewing himself, when he was given several dosages to choose from, from a high of ten parts per million to a low of .5 parts per million, thought he was being safe in selecting a dosage in the lower range. It turned out that he was wrong. The Medical Monopoly, perhaps because it is profiting from the steady increase in deaths among the elderly from drinking fluoridated water, refuses to yield on this question. Fluoridation remains one of the Four Holy Waters of the Church of Modem Medicine.

Ewing and his minions were also aware of Soviet studies showing that fluorides were extremely important in introducing a docile, sheep-like obedience in the general population. It was well known that for years, breeders of purebred bulls had used doses of fluorides to calm their

157

more intractable bulls, making them much safer to handle. The Soviet Union maintained its concentration camps since 1940 by administering increasing dosages of fluorides to the prison population in its vast empire, the Gulag Archipelago, the largest network of concentration camps in the world, and the envy of every bureaucrat in Washington. American totalitarian, alike in every way to their Soviet counterparts, also want all dissension stifled, all resistance ended, and a slave population which pays ever increasing amounts of taxes while having no voice in their own government. The fluoridation campaign has been an important step towards this goal. It may yet prove to have been the crucial step in the complete Sovietization of America. We know that during recent years, the American people have been afflicted with a strange passivity, ignoring each new outrage inflicted upon them by the ravenous federal agents who descend upon their private property in hordes, brandishing automatic weapons which they have no need of using, herding the frightened victims into pens, and degrading them in a manner which no American ever thought to see. This passivity and unwillingness to challenge any authority is merely the first achievement of the fluoridation campaign. This is its initial effect upon the central nervous system. Unfortunately, the further deadly effects upon the kidneys, the cumulative effect on the heart and other organs, as well as the widespread development of new and fast spreading cancer, is yet to come. To hasten this cherished objective, not only are American children being given fluoridated water; they also are told to brush their teeth at least three times a day with heavily fluoridated toothpaste, which contains seven per cent of sodium fluoride. Studies show that children habitually ingest about ten per cent of this solution during each brushing, giving them a daily dose of 30% of the seven per cent solution in the toothpaste.

No doubt this will hasten the Soviet objective. To combat this outrage, one entrepreneur plans to soon market a nonfluoridated toothpaste, which will be called Morgan's Guaranty Toothpaste— "You Can Trust Our Guaranty That This Toothpaste Contains No Harmful Fluorides."

The source of much of this substance is the Aluminum Company of America, a five billion dollar a year enterprise. Its present chairman is Charles W. Parry, a director of the supposedly "right wing" think tank, American Enterprise Institute, of which Jeane Kirkpatrick is the most highly touted member, and principal ornament. The former chairman and still director, of ALCOA, William H. Krome George, is an active director of the well- publicized United States USSR Trade and Economic Council, which is intended to rescue the Soviet Union from economic oblivion.

George is also a director of a number of leading defense companies such as TRW, Todd Shipyards, International Paper, and the Norfolk and Southern Railway. ALCOA's president is William B. Renner, who is a director of the Shell Oil Company, a firm now controlled by the Rothschild interests. Other directors of ALCOA are William R. Cook, chairman of the Union Pacific Railroad, the base of the Harriman fortune; Alan Greenspan, now chairman of the Federal Reserve Board of Governors, whose action in raising the interest rate a few days after he took office precipitated Black Monday, the worst stock market crash in American history. Greenspan's name is not familiar to most Americans, although it should be; he was the chairman of a Special Commission on Social Security, which finagled a horrendous increase in the amount of withholding tax on every working American. Greenspan was able to do this because he was a highly paid Wall Street "consultant," meaning that he could juggle figures to come up with whatever result the Rockefeller Monopoly desired. He conducted a specious campaign to persuade the American people that the Social Security program was bankrupt, when in fact it had reserve funds of $22 billion, plus $25 billion which Congress had borrowed directly from the system, and which was a collectible asset. Greenspan also based his demand for a huge increase in the withholding tax, which was nothing but a tax, on a projected 9.6% increase in the inflation rate, when in fact it was only a 3.5% increase. The alarmed public, frightened by President Reagan's absurd claims that the principal beneficiaries of the Social Security System were the idle rich, was hoodwinked into dropping its objections to the increase in tax. However, actual figures on hand at that time showed that only 3% of the elderly had incomes above $50,000 a year, which in itself was hardly a princely sum in these days of inflation, an inflation which itself was largely created by the government's fiscal policies. Greenspan was the star of the great Social Security "crisis" of 1983, shrewdly capitalizing on the propaganda barrage that the Social Security System was rapidly going broke. His first finding was that Social Security funds would be in the red from $150 to $200 billion by 1990; at the same time, he was telling his high-paying corporate clients it would be only one-third of that sum. The final increase was what he had told his clients. He also "forecast" that the consumer price index would rise to 9.2% by 1985; at the same time, he was informing his corporate clients it would be only one-third of that figure. The actual increase was 3.6%. This performance earned Greenspan a prestigious position as partner of J. P. Morgan Company. He is now chairman of the Federal Reserve Board of Governors. The New Republic defined the function of this body on January 25, 1988 stating plainly, "The Federal Reserve Board protects the interests of the rich." No one has yet challenged that statement. Greenspan is also a director of the giant media conglomerate, Capital Cities ABC Network, as well as being a trustee of the reputedly right wing think tank, Hoover Institution, which furnished the powerhouse behind the "Reagan Revolution," and which is dominated by the Trotskyite League for Industrial Democracy, a Rockefeller funded agitprop group.

The vice chairman of ALCOA is Forrest Shumway, who is also a director of Transamerica, Ampex Corporation, Garrett Corporation, Mack Trucks, The Wickes Companies, Gold West Broadcasters, United California Bank, and Natomas, Inc.; a heady mix of banking interests, heavy industry, and media holdings, which is typical of the monopolists today; they have found the best modus operandi is to control the media, banking and defense industries in a giant combine. Other directors of ALCOA are Paul H. O'Neill, who is a member of the influential Board of Visitors at Harvard University, president of International Paper, and director of the National Westminister Bank, one of England's "Big Five." O'Neill was Chief of Human Resources for the U.S. Government from 1971-77; Paul H. Miller, senior adviser to the prestigious First Boston Investment Group, director of Celanese Corporation, Cummins Engine, Congoleum Corporation, Seamans Bank for Savings, New York, and Ogilvy & Mather, Inc., one of the nation's leading advertising firms; Franklin H. Thomas, the token black who was U.S. Attorney for New York, and then was named head of the Ford Foundation; he is also a director of Citicorp, Citibank, Allied Stores and Cummins Engine; Sir Arvi Parbo, an Australian tycoon who is chairman of the Western Mining Company; he is also director of Zurich Insurance, the second largest firm in Switzerland, Munich Reinsurance, and Chase Manhattan Bank; Nathan Pearson, who for many years has been the financial guardian of the Mellon family, handling their major investments; John P. Diesel, president of the giant conglomerate Tenneco; he is also a director of US—USSR Trade & Economic Council with Armand Hammer, and director of First City Bancorp, one of the three Rothschild banks in the United States; John D. Harper, director of Paribas New York, Metropolitan Life and chairman of Coke Enterprises and other fuel companies; John A. Mayer, director of H. J. Heinz Company, the Mellon Bank and Norfolk and Western Railway—his son, John, Jr., is general manager of the Morgan Stanley bankers in England, and vice president of Morgan Guaranty International.

Thus we see that the origin of the sodium fluoride controversy stems from close allies of the Chase Manhattan Banks and other Rockefeller interests.

The operation of the aluminum trust has given rise to a new epidemic in the United States. Two and one half million Americans are currently afflicted with a strange, incurable disease called Alzheimer's disease. Its victims now require more than $50 billion worth of medical care each year, and the prognosis always grows darker, due to the progressive nature of this illness. It strikes the neurotransmitters of the brain, which, as has already been noted, are adversely affected by fluoride; however, the principal agent seems to be the accumulation of aluminum deposits on the principal nerves of the brain. About 70% of the costs of this illness is borne by the families of the afflicted, because most Medicare and private health insurance programs refuse to pay it. The Medical Monopoly has been frantically trying to find some other agent in this disease, spending millions to study such factors as genetic predisposition, slow virus, environmental toxins, and immunologic changes, despite the fact that its origins have been traced to the large amounts of aluminum which most Americans began ingesting with their food since the 1920s. Alzheimers is now causing more than 100,000 deaths annually, and is the fourth leading cause of adult death in the United States, yet, significantly, there has been no national foundation such as the American Cancer Society or the Arthritis Foundation to investigate its causes, because the Medical Monopoly already knows the answer.

Alzheimer's growing incidence was at first dismissed as "growing old"; later it was diagnosed as "premature senility" (it often strikes in the mid fifties). These were the men and women who had grown up in America during the 1920s, a period when the traditional cast iron and earthenware cooking vessels were almost universally replaced by the more modern, and seemingly more convenient, aluminum cookware. The present writer's parents both grew up on farms in rural areas of Virginia. Their food, almost entirely home grown, was prepared in iron pots over wood-fuelled cookstoves. Those Americans born after 1920 had their food prepared in aluminum pots, which were usually heated over gas flames, later electric. This writer's mother often remarked that food cooked over gas flame never tasted like food cooked over wood fires. The reason is that the combustion of poisonous fuel inevitably releases some toxins into the air, and into the food. Electric heat is also said to materially affect food, because of the electric vibrations given off by the heat.

By the 1930s, American housewives had learned that it was potentially dangerous to leave many foods in aluminum pots for more than a few minutes. Greens, tomatoes, and other vegetables, were known to discolor and became poisonous in a short time.

Tomatoes could actually pit and corrode the interior of the aluminum pots in a short time; many foods turned the pots black. Strangely enough, no one took these obvious warning signs as an indication that cooking food in aluminum pots even for a few minutes might produce unfortunate results. It is now known that cooking any food in an aluminum pot, particularly with fluoridated water, quickly forms a highly poisonous compound. Dr. McGuigan's testimony in a famous court hearing on aluminum effects, the Royal Baking Powder case, revealed that extensive research had shown that boiling water in aluminum pots produced hydro-oxide poisons; boiling vegetables in aluminum also produced a hydro-oxide poison; boiling an egg in aluminum produced a phosphate poison;

boiling meat in an aluminum pot produced a chloride poison. Any food cooked in aluminum containers would neutralize the digestive juices, produce acidosis, and ulcers. Perhaps the use of aluminum pots produced the widespread indigestion in America, which then necessitated the ingesting of large amounts of antacids containing even more aluminum!

After consuming food cooked in aluminum pots over a period from twenty to forty years, many Americans began to experience serious memory loss; their mental capacities then deteriorated rapidly, until they were totally unable to fend for themselves or to recognize their spouses of many years. It was then found that concentrations of aluminum in certain areas of the brain had caused permanent deterioration of brain cells and nerve connections; the damage was not only incurable; it was also progressive and not responsive to any known treatment. This epidemic was soon known as Alzheimer's disease. Seven per cent of all Americans over 65 have now been diagnosed as having this disease. Many others have not been diagnosed; they are simply dismissed as senile, incompetent or mentally ill.

Dr. Michael Weiner and other physicians have found that the epidemic has been caused, not only by the aluminum cookware, but by the daily increasing ingestion of aluminum from many products in common household usage. The insatiable marketers of aluminum have annually expanded its use in many products, whose consumers have no idea that they are ingesting any type of aluminum. Women's douches now contain solutions of aluminum, which introduces it directly into the system. The most widely used painkillers such as buffered aspirin contain impressive quantities of aluminum; Ascriptin A/D (Rorer) has 44 mg. of aluminum per tablet; Cama (Dorsey) has 44 mg. of aluminum per tablet. However, the largest single source of aluminum occurs with the daily ingestion of widely prescribed and nonprescription antacid products for stomach upsets.

Amphojel (Wyeth) has 174 mg per dose of aluminum hydroxide; Alternagel (Stuart) has 174 mg of aluminum hydroxide per dose; Delcid (Merrel National) 174 mg aluminum per dose; Estomil-M (Riker) 265 mg of aluminum per dose; Mylanta II (Stuart) 116 mg aluminum per dose. A study of current victims of Alzheimer's would probably find that most of them, on their physicians' advice, had been ingesting large amounts of these antacids daily for years.

Nonprescription antidiarrhoeal drugs also contain significant amounts of aluminum; Essilad (Central) has 370 mg of aluminum salts per ml; Kaopectate Concentrate (Upjohn) has 290 mg aluminum per ml.

Aluminum ammonium sulfate is widely used as a buffer and neutralizing agent by manufacturers of cereals and baking powder. Aluminum Potassium Sulfate, known as aluminum flour or aluminum meal, is widely used in baking powder and clarifying sugar.

The annual use of sodium aluminum phosphate has now reached the amount of 19 million kilograms per year; it is used in large amounts in cake mixes, frozen dough, self-rising flour, and processed foods, in an average amount per product of from three to three and one-half per cent. Some 300,000 kg. of sodium aluminum sulfates are used in household baking powders each year, averaging from twenty-one to twenty-six per cent of the bulk of these products.

Aluminum wrap is now everywhere; toothpaste is packaged in tubes lined with aluminum; there are aluminum seals on many food and drink products; and soft drinks everywhere are now packaged in aluminum cans. While the amount of aluminum ingested on any given day from all of these sources may be infinitesimal, the parade of products coated with or mixed with aluminum available on a daily basis is frightening. Its effects are the equivalent to that of a slow virus, as the metal accumulates at vital points in the system, particularly in the human brain. Thus the number of Alzheimer's victims is probably outnumbered by the number of potential victims, who will later be afflicted with its terrible symptoms.

CHAPTER 6

WHITHER AIDS?

The most talked-about medical phenomena of the 1980s is AIDS, the "acquired immune deficiency syndrome." The name is of some interest. First of all, it is said to be "acquired," presuming some action on the part of the victim in coming down with this disease. Second, it results in or is characterized by an "immune deficiency," meaning that the human system, loses the ability to fight against and overcome these inimical presences. The result is that the system becomes prey to a variety of infections, some of which will be fatal. The prevalence of these infections occurs through two dominant illnesses, Kaposi's sarcoma, evidenced by large sores on the skin, and a form of pneumonia. It is noteworthy that pneumonia, which had been a fatal disease, had largely been conquered. It had been called "the old man's friend," because it took off many elderly persons who presumably no longer had a desire to live.

The class of infections which have become widespread through what is called AIDS were first recognized by physicians, veterinarians and biologists about fifty years ago. At that time, many sheep in Ireland were afflicted by a killer epidemic called Maedi- Visma. Biologists determined that Maedi-Visma was caused by a new class of viruses. Because of the time they required to become virulent, these viruses were called "slow viruses." The advent of these slow viruses presages a new era in the medical history of mankind. Human beings prior to this time have not been affected by slow viruses, although they have been found among animals being transmissible among monkeys and apes. Slow viruses are also a type known as "retroviruses." When they enter an infected cell, they assimilate into the genetic structure of the cell, apparently during the cell process of mitosis, or cell division, such division being a normal process of healthy growth. Mitosis is one of the two alternatives which face every cell in the human body; either it divides and grows through mitosis as a life process, or it submits to viral replication and resultant cell death as part of a disease process. Thus we find at the crux of the AIDS problem the ultimate question of the life or death of the entire organism. This is why AIDS, once it reaches the virulent stage, is said to be incurable, resulting in the death of the host body.

In a healthy body, some ten million cells are dying every second; at this same second, they are usually replaced by the body process. Such immediate replacement cannot be orchestrated by the usual body processes of genetic information theories, chromosomes, enzymes or nerve impulse signals. The instantaneous nature of the process requires that it be commanded by bioradiation phenomena. These are triggered by coherent ultraweak photon emissions from living tissues of varying wavelengths. These photon emissions, according to their wavelengths, control biological functions which are in constant activity, such as photorepair, photoaxism, photoperiodic clocks, mitosis, and multiphoton events. Ultraweak photon emissions from living cells exhibit a spectral distribution from infrared (900 nm) to ultraviolet (200 nm). This photon intensity correlates with the conformational states of DNA, during which activity the spectral intensities of biophotons amount to magnitudes of some 10/40 magnitude times higher than those of thermal equilibrium at physiological temperatures. The biomolecule with the highest information density, DNA, seems to be the source of biophoton regulatory radiation, functioning as an "exciplex" laser, and comparing favorably with the fields of man-made lasers.

Thus the problem of AIDS brings us to the most basic properties of cell function. The ability of the living cell to respond to microwaves without discernible variation in temperature apparently indicates a nonthermal mechanism like an activated crystal. Thus AIDS may help us in understanding the tuning mechanism of cells, which indicate its state of health or disease and thus improve our understanding of all diseases affecting the organism. A wide ranging study of living cells, from primitive bacteria to those of man, shows that these cells produce natural alternating current (AC) fields which in frequency ranges lower than 100 Mhz, show maximal electrical oscillation at or near mitosis. Here again, tuned systems are triggering biological actions in a manner which is not yet fully understood. Thus the death of Rock Hudson, one of Hollywood's most promiscuous homosexual psychopaths, may lead to the fortunate result of inspiring new breakthroughs in our understanding of the most basic cell functions. Unfortunately, the cancer profiteers and Medical Monopoly insist on treating AIDS as a malfunction of the cell itself, which, of course, calls for the "magic bullet," the chemotherapy which will be provided at a price by the Drug Trust. In fact, chemotherapy attacks the immune system, thus increasing the fatality of the disease. The Establishment approach is to attack the virus, not to aid the system in overcoming it, thus not only bypassing the immune system which is already under attack from this disease, but actually aiding in its conquest.

There have been repeated claims that AIDS is actually a man made virus; it seems to have been unknown prior to 1976, when mild traces of it were discovered in African blood banks. Available evidence indicates that it then began spreading throughout Africa, and subsequently to the United

States, during the mid 70s. A possible reference to this or some other created virus appears in the *WHO Bulletin*, v.47, page 251 in 1972. "An attempt should be made to see if viruses can in fact exert selective effects on immune function. The possibility should be looked into that the immune response to the virus itself may be impaired if the infecting virus damages, more or less selectively, the cell responding to the virus."

Carlton Gadjuske, National Institute of Health director at Ft. Detrick, noted, "In the facility I have a building where more good and loyal Communists, scientists from the USSR and mainland China work, with full passkeys to all the laboratories, than there are Americans. Even the Army's infectious disease unit is loaded with foreign workers not always friendly nationals."

This fuels speculation that such a virus could have been created by alien and unfriendly scientists working in the heart of our own defense laboratories, whether as a plan to decimate our population, or as one more step towards ultimate world domination.

From 1976 to 1981, AIDS was almost exclusively publicly identified as a disease of homosexuals; thus the general population felt no alarm at problems confined to a relatively small group. The few non-homosexuals who came down with AIDS acquired it from public blood banks, through homosexuals who had sold their blood. AIDS was then termed "gay cancer" by doctors who informed patients they had the disease. It was usually unmistakable because of large purplish blotches which disfigured the skin, proof of the presence of Kapsi's sarcoma. At this time, many doctors believed the disease originated in the peculiar physical factors of homosexual activity, with considerable evidence pointing to the use of fatty lubricants in rectal intercourse. These lubricants, introduced into the intestinal area in this unusual manner, apparently provided a fertile breeding ground for the onslaught of the infection. Dr. Lawrence Burton, a noted cancer specialist, raised the question, "What effect does repeated and sustained introduction of lubricants into the anal cavity have upon the immune system?" It was noted that this caused immune depression in test animals. Burton's attorney, W. H. Moore, suggested that hydrogenated fats, either consumed orally or used anally, could cause AIDS. This again brings us back to the role which nutrition plays in any disease, such as the victims of atomic radiation in Japan; those on traditional low fat diet suffered substantially fewer fatalities than those on the modern high fat diet. This also raises again the question of hydrogenated fats and their possible deleterious effect upon the human system, either heated, which produces dangerous chemical changes, or ingested cold.

The initial reaction of many homosexuals, on being informed that they had AIDS, was what has been termed by psychologists, "homosexual rage," a dementia in which the patient is possessed by a mad desire for revenge. The phenomenon of this type of "AIDS dementia" has been observed in some 60 per cent of AIDS patients, bolstering some doctors' belief that AIDS is merely a new variant on the ancient syphilis infection. Syphilis often is characterized by paresis, deterioration of the brain until schizophrenia takes over.

Other physicians have related AIDS dementia to toxoplasmosis, a cat-borne parasite which causes the same type of dementia which afflicts patients with AIDS. The problem with pursuing any of these leads is that not only is the Medical Monopoly waiting in the wings to reap more billions of dollars in profits from this new epidemic, but the civil libertarians are forestalling investigations of AIDS by defending the "privacy" of its victims. Like other groups which either have offended society or have purposefully cut themselves off from what is termed "society," homosexuals have developed a fanatical group loyalty. Many homosexual activists see in AIDS one more representation of the fundamental differences which create an insurmountable barrier between themselves and other humans. As such, they are exploiting it and perhaps are reluctant to see any solution to AIDS.

This group loyalty has manifested itself in a telling way, the determination of many homosexuals with AIDS to infect as many people as possible, not only through greatly extending their already voluminous sexual contacts, but also by infecting others through their bartered blood. In Los Angeles, a James Markowski, who was then in the final stages of AIDS, was arrested June 23, 1987 for selling his blood to the Los Angeles Plasma Production Associates. He admitted that he wanted to infect as many people as possible before he died. On January 7, 1987, a notorious homosexual activist, Robert Schwab, who was also dying of AIDS, made a public appeal to all his confreres, that "gay males" should immediately give blood if they had been diagnosed as having AIDS. "Whatever action is required to get national attention is valid," he declared. "If that includes blood terrorism, so be it." It was noted that following Schwab's widely advertised public appeal, blood donations increased by a dramatic three hundred per cent in New York and San Francisco, the two queenly centers of American homosexuality.

None other than Rock Hudson, when he was informed that he had AIDS, was overcome with "homosexual rage." He immediately launched on a frenetic campaign to infect as many people as possible, concentrating on teen-agers who had no idea of the dangers they were facing. In his insane determination to leave this world in a sexual Gotterdammerung, Hudson must have infected dozens, if not hundreds, of unsuspecting youths. Even today, lawsuits are still pending against his estate, as a result of his orgy of fear and hate.

While the Rock Hudsons were dying their slow and agonizing deaths, most members of the American public viewed them with a mixture of approbation and contempt. There was no fear, because as yet there was no indication of peril to the population at large.

However, as early as September 16, 1983, at a health conference in Washington, D.C. the question was raised by Dr. John Grauerholz, "Will AIDS Become Another Bubonic Plague?" The conference supplied the finding that AIDS "can be the harbinger of a series of holocaustal epidemics." On September 26, 1985, Dr. William Haseltine of Harvard Medical School reported that an estimated ten million Africans were now infected with the AIDS virus. However, government authorities here continued to assure the public that AIDS was limited to four groups, homosexuals, Haitians, intravenous drug users and blacks. Since most American citizens would never come into direct contact with any of these groups, a fetid subunderclass which existed in its own twilight world of filth and degeneracy, it seemed that the AIDS epidemic would never become a threat to the American middle class.

The government agency, the Center for Disease Control in Atlanta, the heroes of the Great Swine Flu Massacre, now did their best to keep the American people in the dark as to a possible spread of AIDS. They issued periodic ukases to the effect that AIDS could not be spread by insects; AIDS could not be contracted by kissing, although they admitted that the AIDS virus was present in saliva; and other reassurances whose scientific validity seems to have been taken directly from the pages of Grimm's Fairy Tales. Even so, CDC estimated that by 1988, from one to one and a half million Americans would be infected with the AIDS virus;

there were already 5,890 members of the U.S. Army who were infected with AIDS. Dr. David Axelrod, Commissioner of Health for the State of New York, solemnly warned that all those who had the AIDS virus were doomed, "Virtually all those infected are doomed."

Dr. John Seale, of Richmond, Virginia presided at a conference June 11, 1987, in which he stated positively, that "AIDS is not a sexually transmitted disease. It is a contagious disease which is also transmitted in blood." He denounced the Surgeon General of the United States, Dr. Everett Koop, for deliberately spreading disinformation about the disease, claiming that joining Koop in this campaign of "scientific disinformation" were Sir Donald Acheson, Chief Medical Officer of the United Kingdom; Dr. Halfdan Mahler, director general of the World Health Organization; Dr. Robert Gallo of the National Institute of Health; and Prof. Viktor Zhdanov, director of the Ivanovsky Institute of Virology in Moscow.

Dr. Seale was not the first to point the finger at Dr. Gallo, resident scientist of the National Institute of Health, who was famed as having discovered the humano-immunio-deficiency virus, HIV, which he claimed was the cause of AIDS. After Gallo's discovery, the NIH, which doles out funds for research on AIDS as well as many other categories, consistently denied funds to any scientist whose work failed to bear out Gallo's claim. President Reagan then appointed a Special Presidential Commission on AIDS, which was intended to solve the problem. It tried to do so by meeting in great secrecy, and by meeting without a quorum, so that no notes could be taken of the proceedings. Admiral James D. Watkins was head of these meetings, which came in for much criticism, merely because the American public wanted to know what was being accomplished.

One of the researchers who was to come into conflict with Dr. Gallo over the "HIV" controversy is Dr. Peter Duesberg, professor of virology at the University of California at Berkeley. Duesberg is also a member of the National Academy of Sciences. He had been brought to Gallo's own laboratory to work under a fellowship grant. After studying HIV in the same laboratory where Gallo had claimed to have made his monumental findings, Dr. Duesberg concluded that the HIV virus did not meet the standard criteria required of a disease-causing agent. He published his findings in the medical journal, *Cancer Research*, in March 1987," and sat back to wait for Dr. Gallo to justify his conclusions. Both he and the editor of *Cancer Research*, Dr. Peter McGee, were amazed when Dr. Gallo made no reply, either then or in the ensuing months. Dr. Gallo also refused to return telephone calls seeking to elicit some reaction to Duesberg's findings. Apparently it was one of those famous "Fact or Fiction" "researches" in which Dr. Gallo had claimed to pinpoint the HIV virus as the sole cause of AIDS. This sort of thing occurs more often than anyone realizes in the academic and scientific world, which is riddled with petty jealousies, calculated deceit, and denial of funds to anyone who might expose their fake research. As we mentioned earlier, most scientists, when asked for their research notes, usually respond that they have been "accidentally burned." Whether anyone has ever seen any of Dr. Gallo's work isolating the HIV virus is not known. However, he has since moved to cut off any further studies of the HIV virus.

Dr. Harvey Baily, research editor of the medical journal *Bio/Technology*, had organized a White House workshop on the subject, "How Does HIV Cause AIDS?" It was to be cohosted by Jim Warner, a senior analyst for domestic policy at the White House. It was expected that Dr. Gallo would attend this conference and present some substantiation of his claims. Warner had already become very skeptical of

Gallo after reviewing Dr. Duesberg's findings. But Gallo never appeared. Instead, the White House Conference, which was scheduled for January 19, 1988, was abruptly cancelled without explanation. Hundreds of millions of dollars continue to be awarded each year to pursue Gallo's questionable claim that the HIV virus causes AIDS. However, no funds are awarded to those who wish to challenge his claims.

Dr. Duesberg has had some interesting experiences since he unwittingly challenged one of the nation's leading bureaucratic scientists. The Presidential Committee on the HIV Virus Epidemic invited him to a special meeting in New York, which was covered by the *Wall Street Journal* scientific writer Katie Leishman. A staff member of this meeting admitted that Duesberg was invited to appear "to discredit him." This goal was thwarted when none of the members of the Presidential Commission could answer any of Dr. Duesberg's findings. They consoled themselves by sharply reprimanding him for having challenged Gallo's work. Dr. William Walsh, who is president of Project Hope, and perennial standard bearer of Establishment values, strongly admonished Duesberg, "Don't confuse the public. Don't confuse the poor people suffering from this disease." Duesberg was himself confused by this approach, as he had never sought to confuse anyone. He had merely pursued a scientific approach which brought into disrepute the leading government scientist. If this upset a Presidential Commission, whose sole function seemed to be to protect Dr. Gallo, this could hardly be Dr. Duesberg's fault. As we commented, the entire imbroglio typifies what passes for serious scientific work in America.

Ms. Leishman characterized the episode as that of "instant orthodoxy which resists review."

Meanwhile, due to the lack of real scientific verification of any single cause, a number of theories about the origin of AIDS have sprung up. These range from the previously mentioned suggestion that it is a new variation on the syphilis spirochete, to a variation of hepatitis virus, which has been endemic for some years, to its kinship with the Epstein-Barr virus, a member of the Herpes Viradae. This is probably the most widely disseminated human virus today, affecting some 95% of the world's population. It is usually transmitted through saliva. Young people come down with it as infectious mononucleosis; its consequences include hepatitis and spelnomegaly, with complications of Reye's syndrome, Guillain- Barre syndrome, Bell's Palsy, and chronic fever and fatigue. Its effects are often mistaken by physicians for multiple sclerosis, Hodgkins disease, leukemia and lupus.

Dr. Stephen Caizza of New York is one of those who identify AIDS as the latest manifestation of syphilis, a logical determination, in view of the fact that it occurs frequently among very promiscuous homosexuals and prostitutes. During the first quarter of 1987, recorded cases of syphilis jumped by twenty-three per cent, the largest increase in a decade. Dr. Peter Duesberg is so positive that there is another agent for AIDS that he has offered to be publicly injected with the AIDS virus. Chuck Ortleb voices another widely held concept, that AIDS is but one variation of the widely encountered chronic-fatigue syndrome, the Epstein-Barr syndrome, which is now worldwide. Other researchers are certain that AIDS is merely one more consequence of the Great Swine Flu Massacre, when the population was injected with the "swine flu" vaccine.

Correlations between AIDS and the real "swine flu," that is, a version of this disease which has been observed among swine, have now been established. Other researchers have blamed a more dramatic or accidental variation of a hepatitis serum which was widely distributed a few years ago. However, none of these theories can compare in narrative value with "the green monkey" theory.

According to this theory, which had long been a favorite explanation advanced by the government propaganda group, the Center for Disease Control, for years a tribe of little green monkeys has roamed in Central Africa. Showing little fear of humans, they have often strayed into native villages. These green monkeys carry in their bloodstream a type of the AIDS virus, to which they are seemingly immune. However, the little green monkeys have either bitten native women or had intercourse with them, depending on which story you wish to believe; the native women's systems then activated the AIDS virus, and later infected their husbands, who then went to Haiti, where they were paid to perform as male prostitutes by members of the American homosexual population who frequently visited Haiti for amusement. These homosexuals then returned to New York infecting the New York community, and commuting to San Francisco, where they spread the disease on the West Coast. This scenario is claimed to have taken place within a few weeks, from green monkey to homosexuals dying with AIDS in San Francisco; however, most researchers believe the disease took quite a few years to reach its present epidemic stage.

A response to the AIDS epidemic was made difficult by the fact that it was confined to the homosexuals, poor blacks, and intravenous drug users, who were known by the slogan "Nothing degenerate is alien to me." The disease became prevalent at the same time that the homosexual movement was emerging as a powerful political force. Allying themselves with blacks, militant homosexuals for all practical purposes took over the Democratic Party, to the dismay of active heterosexuals like Senator Teddy Kennedy. The traditional leaders of the Democratic Party now began to fear publicity about AIDS as originating from the Republican Party, which could pose as "the party of sexual normality." There is little doubt that the conquest of the Democratic Party by the wackos, wresting it away from its longstanding Mafia control, was a boon to the Republicans. The result was that the Democrats fought desperately to keep AIDS in the closet, battling any proposals for AIDS testing or other government measures to control its spread. In San Francisco, a plan to close the bathhouses, the nation's most famous homosexual bordellos, had originated with some of the more frightened homosexuals, who had already seen their "lovers" wither away and die from the disease. Their suggestion was met with a chorus of outrage from the hard-core homos, who were loyally supported by San Francisco's political leaders. It had long been established that the homosexual vote now provided the crucial swing vote needed for victory, in San Francisco, and they were not about to give up their political power. On the national level, government efforts to deal with AIDS have been limited to pathetic and laughable programs to hand out free condoms and free drug needles to the suicidal fringe among the degenerates. In fact, by these tactics, government agencies themselves became official sponsors of homosexual degeneracy and use of narcotics, a strange development for the upholders of the statutes. Reflecting the government's new and more enlightened approach, Bird's Florist, in the nation's capital, celebrated Valentine's Day, 1988 by offering a Valentine Special, consisting of a dozen American Beauty Roses, and a dozen condoms. The package, which was called "The Safe Sex Bouquet," was received with enthusiasm by the government bureaucracy.

Throughout this epidemic, the government has done virtually nothing, while AIDS continues to spread. The Center for Disease Control, in Jimmy Carter's backyard, had continued to be dominated by old line Democratic politicians; any cooperation with the "fascist" regime of

Ronald Reagan was refused. From the outset of the AIDS epidemic, the Center for Disease Control has fought a desperate rearguard action to conceal or play down the epidemic. In the summer of 1985, CDC authorities flatly refused to consider head lice or pubic lice as possible transmitters of the AIDS virus. CDC staff members rejected the idea with horror, lisping that the very notion was "impracticable" and "frightening." In fact, it is well known that many viruses are carried by insects, especially arboviruses, "arthpod-borne-viruses"; some five hundred of these arboviruses have now been identified. Some researchers are certain that the bedbug is one of the principal carriers of the AIDS virus, which is spreading so rapidly throughout Africa; the bedbug is found in almost every African hut. Scientists now believe that mosquitoes, the tsetse fly, the lion ant, and black beetles, may also be transmitting the AIDS virus in Africa. This offers a rational explanation for the rapid spread of AIDS in many different African countries. None of these insects can be found in all African countries, but one or more are present in large numbers in every region of Africa.

In 1900, Dr. Walter Reed proved that the Aedes aegypti mosquito was the vector for yellow fever. It is now known that some monkeys do carry an AIDS type of virus, but as Dr. Duesberg discovered, the HIV virus, to which Dr. Gallo of NIH attributes sole responsibility for AIDS infection, is only present in about half of all AIDS cases, a factor which Dr. Gallo forbears to explain. The question is, what is the infecting agent in the other half of the AIDS cases, or as Dr. Duesberg states, the HIV virus is not the infecting agent in any of them. If this is the case, then the massive government testing programs for the presence of the HIV virus are a multi-million dollar hue and cry after false trails.

Although the Center for Disease Control has continued to insist that poverty, environment, and insects all have absolutely nothing to do with AIDS transmission, an advertisement appeared May 1987 in *Science* magazine seeking a research entomologist who would study "the possible role of biting anthropods in transmitting human immuno-deficiency (AIDS) virus. Apply to the Center for Disease Control."

The perils of offending preconceived theories about AIDS continue to dog researchers. When the Institute of Tropical Medicine presented the results of research it had concluded there, and which indicated there was an arboviral connection to AIDS, the University of Michigan, under considerable pressure from the Center for Disease Control, promptly cut off all of their funding. At Oxford, on August 25, 1986, Prof. Jean-Claude Cermann of Paris' Pasteur Institute reported that AIDS had been found in African insects; the virus had been isolated in mosquitoes, cockroaches, ants and tsetse flies. This was a direct contradiction to the claims of the CDC that the AIDS virus could not be carried by mosquitoes or any other insects.

California physician Bruce Halstead, M.D., states that modern medicine has no cure for AIDS, cancer or radiation sickness. He also points out that his research establishes that the AIDS virus is capable of one trillion mutations. Meanwhile, AIDS patients who are being treated by onocologists (cancer specialists) are reported to be dying at a much greater rate than AIDS patients who are being treated by holistic methods. Many of them are surprising medical statisticians by surviving longer than the two year time span allotted after the diagnosis of the disease. One forty year old patient in San Francisco, Dan Turner, is now the longest surviving victim of AIDS. He says he was infected during a trip to New York in June 1981, and on February 12, 1982, he was informed by a physician that he had "gay cancer," after developing the unmistakable symptoms of Kaposi's sarcoma. He had observed a regimen of Vitamin C, natural foods, meditation, acupuncture, and weight lifting.

Laurence Badgley, M.D., in his ground-breaking work, "Healing AIDS Naturally," offers a number of treatments, a typical one having shown good results with a vegetarian diet of vegetables, vitamins, wheat grass, juice and herbs, which is accompanied by eight or nine cloves of raw garlic each day.

While the government fiddles, the American public continues to burn at the thought of being infected with AIDS, a fatal disease. Referees at boxing matches and other blood sports now wear medical gloves, to avoid being infected by spattering blood from the contestants. Court officials don protective clothing such as gloves and surgical masks when forced to appear in court with diseased AIDS victims. These accoutrements arouse rage and horror from civil libertarians, who claim these protective techniques create a "harmful atmosphere" for the AIDS patient. Since he is probably already dying, the argument would seem to be moot.

The established fact that from its outset, the AIDS epidemics was confined to the well-identified groups of homosexuals, Haitians, intravenous drug users, and blacks, has also created a furor at the American Civil Liberties Union, it being a precept of egalitarian society that a disease should not be so bigoted in choosing its victims. In New York State prisons from 1984 to 1986, the toll of AIDS victims was 45% hispanic, 43% black, with 97% of them being intravenous drug users (New York Times, February 7, 1988).

This writer having previously established in "The Curse of Canaan" that homosexuality, from the time of Canaan himself to the present day, has had its origins in pollution of the original root race, the confusion of sexual identity being a direct consequence of the resulting confusion of racial identity, confusing the DNA pattern of the genetic structure, it is hardly surprising to find in Joy Schulenberg's useful book, "Complete Guide to Gay Parenting," Doubleday 1985, that "gay" couples who are white are found to adopt almost exclusively black children. This is unfair to the black adoptees, who, through no fault of their own, will then be exposed to the possibility of contracting AIDS from one or the other of their "gay" foster parents. It would seem that "gay" whites are unwilling to expose other whites to the perils of the "alternative life style."

CHAPTER 7

FERTILIZER

One of the great changes in our world during the last fifty years has been the "green revolution," the so-called agricultural revolution in many parts of the Third World. This revolution was supposed to rapidly bring the Third World countries into the twentieth century, and allow them to compete on an equal basis with the more advanced Western nations. As the twentieth century now recedes into history, it is apparent that this objective has not been achieved. Asian and Latin American countries are offering more competition in the production of finished goods at a much cheaper labor cost, but in agriculture, despite the fact that vast new markets have been created for the Rockefeller chemical operations, the alleviation of poverty, which supposedly was the goal of the "green revolution" remains a chimera. In fact, those areas of the world which have long been marked on the maps as "undeveloped" had no notation of the fact that this was a code word for "unexploited," that is, not yet exploited by the rapacious international conspirators. The only real interest of the financiers is to develop markets for their products which can return a profit. Because most of the Third World countries are unable to pay for goods, a complex system has been developed whereby the American taxpayer sends "aid" to the Third World. He works in a factory to make a tractor; the tractor is then sent to Bolivia, and then a payment for it is extorted from the worker's wages. A further refinement is a system whereby American or international banks "lend" the money to these countries so that they can pay for the goods; the Federal Reserve System then "guarantees" these uncollectible loans with American taxpayers' funds. Once again, the worker has the money extorted from his paycheck to cover the cost of the goods he produces. The framers of the Constitution never envisioned such a development, with the result that when the worker cites the Constitution for relief from the extortion, the judge indignantly throws him into jail for "irrelevant" and "confusing" testimony. The world is now a Gulag Archipelago, run by the ruthless minions of the Rockefeller-Rothschild conglomerate. Its gods are money and power; its only enemy is the advocate of liberty.

The current hero of the Rockefeller interests is Norman Borlaug, who was awarded the Nobel Peace Prize in 1970. An Iowa farmer, Borlaug had been sent to Mexico by the Rockefeller interests in 1944 to develop new types of grain. During his experiments there, he mated 60,000 different species of wheat, resulting in the creation of an all tropical race of dwarfs, double dwarfs and triple dwarfs by 1964. This was hailed as "the green revolution." The resulting "superwheat" produced greater yields, but this was done by "hyping" the soil with huge amounts of fertilizer per acre, the fertilizer being the product of nitrates and petroleum, commodities controlled by the Rockefellers. Huge quantities of herbicides and pesticides were also used, creating additional markets for the Rockefeller chemical empire. In effect, "the green revolution" was merely a chemical revolution. At no point could the Third World nations be expected to pay for the huge amounts of chemical fertilizers and pesticides. This was again taken care of by the system of "foreign aid" which was already in place.

The Rockefeller interests also sent Robert Chandler to the Philippines to develop a "Miracle Rice"; the result was a rice which used three times the previous amount of fertilizer. This rice matured in four months instead of the previous six months, producing three crops a year instead of two. When two Phillippine groups of wealthy entrepreneurs began to contest each other for local spinoffs of the profits of "Miracle Rice," the Rockefellers decided to oust one group, the Marcos combine, replacing it with the Aquino faction, which had close ties to the Chase Manhattan Bank, and which could be depended on to pay interest on loans. As usual, Rockefeller "philanthropy" was closely inter-linked with markets, profits and political control. Modern fertilizer is a petroleum based industry.

At the conclusion of the Second World War, the munitions manufacturers found themselves faced with huge inventories of nitrates. Because of the outbreak of peace, which is always regarded with horror by the philanthropic foundations, new markets had to be found, and quickly, for these commodities. Nitrogen and nitrates were key ingredients in the manufacture of bombs and shells. A comparable peacetime market had to be developed. Following the precept which they had established after the First World War, when the monopolists, faced with a huge supply of leftover chlorine, which had been manufactured at great expense to cause intensive suffering and death, found that the only possible market was to sell it to American communities, who would then pour it into their water supplies, it was decided in 1945 that the only outlet for the huge inventory of nitrates was to put it into the food chain, as fertilizer.

The increasing rate of deaths from heart attacks in the United States for the past fifty years has been ingenuously explained by apologists for the Medical Monopoly as one more illustration of the "fact" that Americans were living longer, their advancing years making them more susceptible to "degenerative" diseases such as cancer and heart trouble. This was the usual copout from the medical establishment, which conveniently ignored important advances in the

American lifestyle. For a number of years during the nineteenth century, epidemics of cholera and typhoid fever had devastated the inhabitants of large American cities, the outbreaks being due to poor sanitation and contamination of the water supply. When the monopolists poured their excess chlorine into the water supplies after the First World War, the result was widely hailed as having ended the epidemics of cholera and typhoid fever. In fact, chlorination had not been responsible for this development. Typhoid fever had been largely due to the contamination of city streets by large quantities of horse droppings, which festered and drew flies.

When it rained, this contamination was washed into the water supply. With the advent of the automobile, and the disappearance of horses from city streets as our main means of transportation, typhoid fever vanished almost overnight. This occurred during the 1920s, when automobiles replaced horses on the streets.

The dumping of this war material into our water supply did have one unforeseen effect. It brought on a new epidemic, an epidemic of heart attacks. The chlorine in the water combined with animal fats in the diet to form a chemical amalgam, which then formed a gummy substance in the arteries; this created a medical condition called atherosclerosis. The buildup of this gummy substance in the arteries gradually interfered with the circulation of the blood, finally closing off the main arteries to the heart, and bringing on the attacks of angina pectoris and coronary heart attacks. Here again, a seeming "advance" in hygiene proved to be yet another boon for the Medical Monopoly, as the offices of the physicians were filled with Americans suffering from heart disease.

At the conclusion of World War II, the monopolists began a concerted effort to dump their surplus nitrates into the American food chain. County agents throughout the

United States were told to advise farmers in their areas to increase their use of fertilizers, herbicides and pesticides. This advice served to make farming even more capital intensive, forcing the farmers to go to the banks to borrow more money, and paving the way for the program of forcing the individual farmers off the land, creating great agricultural monopolies, similar to the Soviet Agricultural Trust. Farmers also borrowed heavily to buy expensive tractors which ran on gasoline, greatly adding to the Rockefeller revenues, and at the same time depriving them of the fertilizer formerly available from their horses. It was hardly coincidental that the banks, which so cheerfully anted up the loans needed by the farmers who faithfully followed the instructions of their county agents, were banks who got their funds from the Federal Reserve System. This monopoly of the nation's money and credit had been planned at a secret meeting of conspirators on Jekyl Island, Georgia in November of 1910, a meeting presided over by Senator Nelson Aldrich, whose daughter had recently married John D. Rockefeller, Jr.

The nutritional value of foods grown in heavily fertilized soil, and the fact that these foods then undergo extensive "processing" to render them more convenient for large scale warehousing, transportation and retailing, has been glossed over by the Medical Monopoly. A protesting voice was heard when Dr. H. M. Sinclair, a leading nutritionist, and head of the Laboratory of Human Nutrition, Magdalen College, Oxford, gave a 1957 World Health Day address, which was reprinted in the *British Medical Journal*, December 14, 1957. Dr. Sinclair recalled that from his earliest days as a medical student, "my clinical teachers could not answer why the expectation of life in this century of the middle-aged man is hardly different from what it was at the beginning of this century, or even a century ago. This means that despite the great advances in medicine— pneumonia almost abolished, tuberculosis comparatively rare, the magnificent advances in surgery, endocrinology, and public health—a middle-aged man cannot expect to live more than four years longer than he could a century ago—and indeed, in Scotland, the expectation of life is now actually decreasing."

In 1893, a German agricultural chemist, Dr. Julius Hensel, wrote in his book "Bread From Stones," "Agriculture has entered into the sign of cancer ... we cannot be indifferent to what kind of crops we raise for our nourishment or with what substances our fields are fertilized. It cannot be all sufficient that great quantities are harvested, but that great quantity must also be of good quality. It is indisputable that by merely fertilizing with marl, i.e., with carbonate of lime, such a large yield may be obtained as to make a man inclined to always content himself with marl, but with such a one-sided fertilization slowly but surely, evil effects of various kinds will develop; these have given rise to the axiom of experience: "Manuring with lime makes rich fathers but poor sons." As our present fine flour, freed from bran, furnished almost entirely devoid of nutrients, we need not wonder at the great number of modern maladies." This was written in 1893, before the Rockefeller interests flooded the world with their petroleum based fertilizers.

To counteract the growing array of inert, nutrition deficient foods, the minions of the Medical Monopoly have not been idle. While conducting wars of attrition against the leading exponents of better nutrition, the Food and Drug Administration and the American Medical Association have valiantly defended the use of chemical fertilizers. The widely circulated AMA magazine, *Today's Health,* found in every public school and library, in September 1958, stated, "Extensive research conducted by the Federal Government has shown that the nutritional value of crops is not affected by the soil of the fertilizers used . . ." This was contradicted by the Rockefeller Foundation's own Dr. Alexis Carrel, who wrote, "Chemical fertilizers, by increasing the abundance of the crops without replacing all the exhausted elements of the soil, have indirectly contributed to change the nutritive value of cereal grains and vegetables. Hens have been compelled by artificial diet and mode of living, to enter the ranks of mass producers. Has not the quality of their eggs been modified? The same question may be asked about milk, because cows are now confined to the stable all year round, and are fed with manufactured provender. Hygienists have not paid sufficient attention to the genesis of diseases. Their studies of conditions of life and diet, and of their effect on the physiological and mental state of modern man, are superficial, incomplete and of too short duration."

Despite the claims of government researchers, the importance of soil is shown by the fact that the proportion of iron in lettuce can vary from 1 mg per hundred to 50 mg per hundred, according to conditions of the soil in which it is grown. The Middle West has long been known as "the goiter belt," because of a widespread deficiency of iodine in the soil. The British Isles, which have been heavily farmed for almost two thousand years, have such deficiencies of minerals in the soil that the British are known the world over for then-bad teeth.

The present system of agricultural chemistry was fathered by Dr. Justus von Liebig, a German chemistry professor who suggested that minerals should be added to the soil and acids added to make them more available to plants. Chemistry agriculture uses soluble chemicals which are either acidic or basic, their final effect being to acidify the soil, while the use of chemical minerals renders the soil useless. It has been suggested that we are still living on the benefits conferred by the last Glacial Age, and that the only way to remineralize the soil is to undergo another Glacial Age, as has previously happened about every 100,000 years.

Dr. W. M. Albrecht, chairman of the Department of Soils at the University of Missouri School of Agriculture, states, "While it has long been common belief that disease is an infliction visited upon us from without, there is a growing recognition that it possibly originates from within because of deficiencies and failure to nourish ourselves completely. Fuller knowledge of nutrition is revealing mounting numbers of cases of deficiency diseases. These tend to be traced, not only to the supplies in the food and supermarket where the family budget may provide them, but a bit further, and closer to their origin, namely, the fertilization of the soil, the point at which all agricultural production takes off. These increasing cases classified as deficiencies are bolstering the truth of that old adage, which told us that 'to be well fed is to be healthy.' "

Many of the strange new diseases which have arisen to plague us in recent years are found to have a nutritional origin. Dr. Josephson identifies myasthenia gravis as an endocrine disorder resulting from a deficiency of manganese, which may be caused either by defective assimilation of manganese or by defective metabolism. The need for chemical fertilizers may have stemmed from a longstanding flaw in the method of farming, the use of the moldbord plow. Edward H. Faulkner, professor at the University of Oklahoma, discovered that the moldbord plow was destroying the fertility of the soil. He counteracted this effect by disking green manure into the surface and eliminating the plow, an instrument which sandwiches virtually all green manure (decaying plant matter and vegetable residue found on the surface of the ground) some six to eight inches below the surface, where it forms a barrier to water, which should rise from the water table. The upper six inches then becomes dry, as the capillary action of water movement is blocked. Plants grown on this plow-depleted soil attract insects, while their vitamin and mineral content is depleted. The plants become sickly and die.

Seeing this result, the farmer then decides that the problem is the lack of some element in the soil, not realizing that it is the plow which has interfered with the capillary action of water in the soil. He then becomes a ready customer for large quantities of chemical fertilizers. One of the principal producers of these fertilizers was the Rockefeller-controlled American Agricultural and Chemical Company. Not surprisingly, one of its directors, John C. Traphagen, was also a director of the Federal Reserve Bank of New York and the Rockefeller Institute of Medicine. A prime mover and director of the American Cancer Society, Traphagen was president of the Bank of New York, and director of the Fifth Avenue Bank. He was also a director of Wyandotte Chemicals, Hudson Insurance, Brokers and Shippers Insurance, Caledonian American Insurance, Foreign Bondholders Protective Association, Sun Insurance, Ltd. (one of the three principal Rothschild firms), Atlantic Mutual Insurance, Eagle Fire Insurance, Norwich Union Fire Insurance, Ltd., International Nickel, Royal Insurance Company, Royal Liverpool Insurance, and many other London insurance firms, most of whom were within the Rothschild orbit.

Also on the board of American Agricultural and Chemical was John Foster Dulles, of the Wall Street law firm, Sullivan and Cromwell; he served as Eisenhower's Secretary of State while his brother Allen was head of the Central Intelligence Agency. Dulles was also a director of International Nickel, Bank of New York, American Banknote Company (which furnished the paper used by the Federal Reserve System to print its paper money, which was backed by paper bonds) and chairman of the Carnegie Endowment for International Peace, of which Alger Hiss was President, director of the New York Public Library, Union Theological Seminary, and the New York State Banking Board. Dulles had been secretary at the Hague Peace Conference in 1907, and served as his uncle's secretary at the Paris Peace Conference in 1918, Robert Lansing, Wilson's Secretary of State. Dulles later served on the Reparations Commission and the Supreme Economic Council with Bernard Baruch in 1919; he attended the Berlin Debt Conference in 1933, and was American delegate to the United Nations in San Francisco when Alger Hiss wrote the United Nations Charter in 1945. Both Dulles and brother Allen had attended a historic conference with Baron Kurt von Schroder and Adolf Hitler in Cologne in 1933, when the Dulles brothers assured Hitler that Wall Street bankers would advance him the money to launch his Nazi regime in Germany.

Also on the board of American Ag & Chem was George C. Clark of the investment bankers, Clark and Dodge; John R. Dillon, chairman of Unexcelled Chemical Company, Lone Start Cement, and was also a theatre tycoon, director of National Theatres, Twentieth Century Fox, Skouras Theatres, and also an aircraft tycoon, as director of Curtiss-Wright and Wright Aeronautical; also on the board was banker Robert Stone, partner of Hayden Stone, director of Rockefeller's Mesabi Iron Ore and Island Greek Coal Company, Punta Alegre Sugar Company, U.S. Envelope, John P. Chase Company, Philadelphia and Norfolk Steamship Company, Amoskeag Company and William Whitmore Company.

Another member of Ag & Chem was Elliott V. Bell, who was also director of the American Cancer Society. He had been a financial writer for the *New York Times* from 1929 to 1939, which gave him entree into the highest financial circles. He became economic adviser to Thomas Dewey in 1940, Supt. of Banks for New York State from 1947-49, director of McGraw Hill, editor of the business magazine *Business-week,* director of Rockefeller's Chase Manhattan Bank, New York Life, New York Telephone Company, Tricontinental Corporation, Revere Copper and Brass and other firms. He also was appointed to the Committee on Social Security Finance for HEW, and trustee of the John S. Guggenheim Foundation, the Roger Straus Foundation. His daughter is a leading New York socialite, Mrs. Thomas Hoving, one of the "beautiful people."

The use of chemical fertilizers caused the protein content of vegetables to drop steadily at the rate of ten per cent a year.

However, the most dangerous effect, and the probable cause of much nutritionally induced disease, was the fact that chemical fertilizer reduced the amount of potassium in the soil, while increasing the amount of sodium. Potassium and sodium are the leaders of the two electrically opposite groups. Inactive potassium in the system precipitates illness, especially cancer. The increased sodium may explain the dramatic increase in the incidence of high blood pressure throughout the United States, because our population is ingesting steadily increasing amounts of sodium from foods grown in chemically fertilized soil, while simultaneously suffering from the effects of steadily declining levels of potassium in the human system. Potassium is especially necessary for the regulation of the heart beat; its lack in the body makes the system prone to sudden heart attacks.

Nutritionists now believe that the use of chemical fertilizers in the soil causes seventy per cent of all anemia in the citizens of the United States, because these fertilizers do not replace iron in the soil, but actually remove it.

The use of chemical fertilizers also accelerated the domination of the world's grain supply by large corporations which are closely affiliated with the Rockefeller interests. In 1919, the largest grain grower in the world was the Montana Farming Corporation. At that time, wheat was selling for a guaranteed price of $2.20 a bushel and the combine was raking in huge profits. Montana's board of directors was headed by J. P. Morgan, whose vast interests in banking, steel and railroads had given no inkling of his desire to become a farmer; Morgan was serving on the Federal Advisory Council of the Federal Reserve Board, representing the New York central banking area. His associates on the board of Montana Farming were Rockefeller's banker, James Stillman of the National City Bank—two of his daughters married two sons of William Rockefeller; Francis Hinckley Sisson, vice-president of the Morgan controlled bank, Guaranty Trust—it is now Morgan Guaranty Trust; Charles D. Norton, whom Morgan placed as President Taft's personal secretary during the Taft presidency. Norton served as president of Morgan's First National Bank (later merged with Rockefeller's National City Bank to form the present banking giant, Citibank). Norton had been one of the original conspirators present at Jekyl Island to secretly draft the Federal Reserve Act. He was a director of Montgomery Ward, Equitable Life, ATT, Tidewater Oil, and the Delaware and Lackawanna Railroad. He was also director of a number of Morgan's favorite charities, the American Red Cross, the Russell Sage Foundation and the Metropolitan Museum. Also on the board of Montana Farming was Charles H. Sabin, a director of Guaranty Trust, Merchants and Metals National Bank, president of the Asia Banking Corporation, American Foreign Securities Corporation, the Mackay Companies, Postal Telegraph and many other firms.

Today, the world grain trade is firmly in the hand of five firms, Cargill, Continental Grain, Louis Dreyfus, Bunge and Andre. These firms have waxed rich and powerful by riding the tide of the supergrains developed by the Rockefeller Trust. They maintain close contact with these interests, and the banking interests of the Rockefellers, relying principally on the Chase Manhattan international network. These firms have also profited from the Rockefeller Foundation's development of hybrid seeds, notably corn. From a commercial standpoint, the attraction of the hybrids is that they cannot reproduce themselves. As a result, the farmer has to ante up the money to buy a new supply of the hybrid seeds each year. Hybrid seeds have another great attraction for the monopolists; they give the parent company, which owns the patent, a monopoly on that particular variety of seed. Thus we have the twin factors of commercial viability and monopoly to give the banks and the Chemical Trust a stranglehold on the American Farmer. Hybrid seeds yield an average increase of twenty to thirty per cent more per acre, which is a strong selling point to the farmer. Likewise the "miracle wheat" which was originated at the International Maize and Wheat Improvement Center at El Butan, Mexico, resulted in the development of a wheat strain which could stand up under the force of lashing rains and tropical storms. It was produced by crossing Mexican wheat with the strains of Japanese dwarfs which had short, tough stems. Norin-10, from the island of Honshu, was hardy enough to stand up under Japanese typhoons. It became the type which made the "green revolution" a reality. After 1960, the Mexican station released a long line of wheats, Nanair 60, for the year 1960, Pitic 62, Penjamo 62, Sonora 64, Lerma Rojo 64, India 66, Siete Cerros 66, Super X 67, Yecoar 70, and Cajeme 71. Although they required intensive fertilization and irrigation, they all could thrive in tropical countries. The Big Five wield enormous political and financial power because of their enormous cash flow, and because so many governments depend on their food supply to maintain political stability. This was demonstrated during what historians now call the Great Soviet Grain Robbery in 1972.

Arranged by Henry Kissinger, longtime Rockefeller stooge from the Chase Manhattan Bank, this deal bailed out the tottering Soviet government, while costing the American taxpayer many billions. In July, 1972, the Soviet Union bought wheat from the United States, in an attempt to compensate for the disastrous incompetence of the Soviet communal system of agriculture. In 1963, Russia had begun a policy of purchasing wheat from abroad by buying 6.8 million tons from Canada for $500 million. To pay for the purchases from the United States in 1972, the Soviet Union was allowed to cover the payment in the following manner; the central bank of Hungary, acting for the Soviet Union, placed an order to sell the dollar short for $20 billion. Secretary of the Treasury, John Connally, then devalued the dollar by ten per cent. The Soviet Union made $4 billion on its short selling of the dollar, and paid for the grain.

Michel Sidona, who had been deeply involved with the Rothschilds and the Hambro family in international financial manipulations, described the process from his prison cell, where he was later found dead. "In its fathomless naivete, the United States has provided the Soviet Union with $4 billion, money that has since doubtless been invested in the destruction of its benefactors; I began to see then that America was the consort of its own ruin. I tell you, in all of history, no power has so blindly armed and succored its enemies as she."

The Soviet grain deal resulted in increasing the price of all food supplies in the United States by twenty per cent. Because of restrictions imposed by Congress on shipping grain in foreign vessels, a measure which had been passed to aid our dwindling maritime fleet, the Soviet grain purchases in 1972 cost the American taxpayer an additional fifty-five million dollars in subsidies to bulk carriers. The American carriers shipped the grain for sixteen dollars a ton, although foreign vessels would have carried it for nine dollars a ton.

To this day, only a few international grain traders and Soviet officials actually know the price charged for forty million tons of grain which the Soviets bought from the United States between 1971 and 1977. Officials at the U.S.

Dept. of Agriculture state that they have no records on the price paid, or whether it was ever paid. Only Henry Kissinger knows, and he is not telling.

The Big Five grain dealers are also heavily involved in currency manipulations, trading vast sums each day in currency futures, because their grain deals cause great fluctuations in the valuation of world currencies. With their inside track, they make huge profits whether the value of the currencies moves up or down. Cargill now has 25% of the world's grain trade; Bunge of Argentina has 20%; Continental Grain began operations during the Napoleonic Wars, supplying grain to both sides; it has 25% of the world grain trade—the present head of the firm, Michel Fribourg, owns 90% of the stock, with his son Rene; Michel Fribourg was a French citizen who joined the U.S. Army Intelligence during World War II; he subsequently became a U.S. citizen; Andre, a Swiss family belonging to a strict sect of Swiss Calvinists who are members of the worldwide and very militant Plymouth Brethren; and Dreyfus, which has twenty per cent of the world grain trade. Dreyfus is now headed by Nathaniel Samuels, who served on President Nixon's team as Under Secretary for Economic Affairs. The chairman of Bunge, Walter Klein, whose office is at One Chase Manhattan Plaza, New York, is a policy-making official of the U.S.-USSR Trade & Economic Council.

CHAPTER 8

CONTAMINATION OF THE FOOD CHAIN

The National Academy of Sciences recently estimated that 15% of the American people are presently afflicted with allergies to one or more chemical products. The study pointed out that we are exposed to more toxic chemicals while inside our homes than when we go out. The chemicals which are found in every home include benzene, which causes leukemia; the common moth spray and mothballs containing para-dichlorobenzene, whose use forms an invisibly but damaging gas in some thirty million American homes; lindane, a common pesticide; chlordane, used for termite control (chlordane has been much in the news lately because of some families who became deathly ill after their homes has been treated by professional termite exterminators; one couple had to move out and totally abandon their home, after inspectors informed them there was no way it could be sufficiently cleansed of the chlordane residues to be habitable). Chloroform compounds are much more common in homes than is popularly realized. The EPA has found that chloroform levels inside of homes was five times greater than outside. Persons taking hot shower baths inside a closed shower curtain are unaware that they are inhaling substantial amounts of chloroform from the steam. Heating the water releases the chlorine in the heavily chlorinated water, which then emerges as a gas while the hot water comes from the nozzle. A daily shower is guaranteed to give you a chloroform high. Formaldehyde is also present in many homes in a number of commonly used compounds.

The daily ingestion of minute portions of any or all of these household chemicals contributes to the development of cancers, as they are sufficiently toxic to become carcinogenic in daily contact. However, Dr. A. Samuel Epstein, a noted cancer authority from the University of Illinois, states that "Food is the single most important route of exposure for humans to synthetic chemicals." Jim Sibbinson estimated that the average American ingests some nine pounds of chemicals in foodstuffs each year, meaning chemicals so toxic that a fraction of an ounce can cause serious illness or death. These chemicals are put into our food chain as additives, preservatives, dyes, bleaches, emulsifiers, antioxidants, flavors, buffers, noxious sprays, acidifiers, alkalizers, deodorants, moisteners, anti-caking and anti-foaming agents, conditioners, curers, hydrolizers, hydrogenators, drying agents, gases, extenders, thickeners, sweeteners, maturers fortifiers, and other agents.

Most Americans are not aware that of the more than five thousand chemical additives in the foods which they eat every day, about one-third are known to be harmless, another third are described by the Food and Drug Administration as "gras," an acronym for "generally recognized as safe," and the other third, almost 2,000 chemicals, are being used in large amounts, even though they have never been adequately tested for possible harmful results. An effort was made to control the use of these chemicals by Rep. James J. Delaney of New York, in 1958. He introduced the Delaney clause, which was enacted into law. It stated that if any food additive is found to induce cancer when ingested by man or animal, it is to be designated unsafe and cannot be used.

The Delaney Committee, which conducted Hearings from 1950 to 1952, listed 704 chemical additives, of which only 428 were known to be safe. The other 276, which continued to be used without any proof that they were safe, meant that the food processors were playing Russian roulette with the American consumer. Even so, it was another six years before the Delaney Amendment became law, requiring testing of these additives. In the ensuing years, some of these chemicals have been dropped in favor of other substances, while others continue to be used without any positive tests to indicate whether they are safe or unsafe. For more than fifty years, food colorings had been made from such poisonous substances as lead, chromium, and arsenic. In any case, the crux of the Delaney Amendment called for the testing of food additives to find whether they caused cancer in man or animal. The catch is that most additives are only tested for toxicity, not for their propensity to cause cancer.

Coumarin, which was a key ingredient of imitation vanilla flavoring, had been in continuous use for seventy-five years before it was found to produce serious liver damage in laboratory animals. An artificial sweetening agent, dulcin, was used as a sugar substitute for fifty years before it was found to produce cancers in test animals. Butter yellow was found to cause cancer of the liver, that is, AB and OB Yellow. Mineral oil, the famous Rockefeller cancer cure of the mid-1800s, which was now used in many salad dressings, was found to prevent the absorption by the body of vitamins and other nutritional needs.

The 1938 Food and Drug Cosmetics Act certified nineteen dyes for use in foods. Since then, three have been decertified, leaving sixteen for use in foods. The label "certified" simply means that it is pure—it offers no clue as to its possible effects on the human system. Dr. Arthur A. Nelson reported that FDA tests in 1957 reported that ten of the thirteen certified dyes then in use had produced cancers when injected under the skin of rats. Science writer, Earl Ubell, estimated that humans would get twice as much of these dyes by mouth as the rats had injected under their skin.

The oil-soluble colors were so poisonous that the rats died before the scientist could see whether any cancer had developed. Nine of the dyes commonly used in foods in the United States are as follows:

Orange No. 1—*used in fish pastes, carbonated beverages, jellies, puddings and many other foods* (now decertified).

Orange No. 2—*Cheese, margarine, candies, exteriors of orange fruit* (now decertified).

Yellow No. 1—*Confectionery, spaghetti and other pastas, baked goods, beverages.*

Yellow No. 3 (Yellow AB)—*Edible fats, margarine, butter, candy.*

Yellow No. 4 (Yellow OB)—*Margarine, butter, candy.*

Green No. 1—*Cordials, candy, bakery goods, soft drinks, jellies, frozen desserts.*

Green No. 2—*Frozen desserts, candies, cakes, jellies, biscuits, cordials.*

Green No. 3—*Bakery products, candies, jellies, desserts.*

Blue No. 1—*Frozen desserts, jellies, puddings, ice cream, candies, cake, icings.*

Yellow AB and Yellow OB, which are known cancer hazards, have been widely used to color margarine and butter. They are made from a dangerous chemical called beta-napth-ylamine. It is notable because it has low toxicity, that is, it is not poisonous in its effect, but it is one of the most carcinogenic substances known. Orange No. 2, Otylazo-2-naphthol, which had been used heavily in United States, the food industry using thousands of pounds of Orange No. 2 annually, was finally discontinued in 1956 when it was found to induce intestinal polyps and cancer in test animals.

White bread, which had long been known to cause brain seizures in dogs, because of the loss of critical nutritional ingredients in processing the beautiful white flour, has in recent years been enriched with a wide variety of vitamins and nutrients. However, a shot of synthetic vitamins, another shot of emulsifier to keep it soft, and the addition of other ingredients, suggests that it might well be produced from a test tube instead of a bakery.

Emanuel Kaplan and Ferdinand A. Dorff, researchers with the Health Department in Baltimore, presented a report, "Exotic Chemicals in Food," which was presented at a meeting of FDA officials. We quote,

"Let us quickly consider the chemical treatment of the various ingredients used in bakery practice. The flour is derived from seeds probably treated for plant disease protection with organic mercurials or similar agents, and the seeds are planted on soil influenced by fertilizers. Selenium (an extremely poisonous mineral substance) may be extracted from the soil. In milling, flour is treated with improvers, oxidizing agents such as persulfate, bromate, iodate and nitrogen tricholoride, which affect protease activity and gluten properties.

"Bleaching agents such as oxides of nitrogen, chlorine and benzoyl peroxide convert the yellow carotenoid pigment to colorless compounds because of alleged consumer desire for white bread.

Vitamins and minerals are added in compulsory 'enrichment.'

Mineral salts may be added to stabilize gas-retaining properties of flour gluten. Cynanide or chlorinated organic compounds may be employed in fumigation of the resulting flour in storage.

"The water used may be chemically purified by means of alum, soda ash, copper sulfate and chlorine. Ammonium salts and other chemicals are employed as yeast nutrients. Chemical leaveners may contain sodium bicarbonate, alum, tartrates, phosphates, starch, and cream of tartar. Fluorine is a possible natural contaminant of the phosphate. Oleomargarine, if used, may have added color, vitamin A, neutralizes, interface modifiers and preservatives; or the margarine may be packed in a preservative-treated wrapper. Mineral oil is frequently used as a dough trough or pan lubricant. Milk or milk products may contain neutralizer and antioxidants. Artificial coal tar color may be used. Stabilizers and thickeners such as gums and treated starches may be employed as fillers. Synthetic flavors used contain glycerine, alcohol or substitute chemicals as solvents for a variety of alcohols, esters, acids, and ketones, and may contain saccharine. *(Ed. Note: This would probably be replaced today by aspartame, an artificial sweetener widely used, which is said to cause brain seizures.)* Spices may be natural spices subjected to fumigants or solvent-extracted spice essences. Mold inhibitors such as calcium propionate may be employed and the final product may be contaminated on the store shelf with insecticidal powders such as sodium fluoride."

Since this report was delivered in the 1950s, many new chemicals have come onto the market, whose properties may be either more or less dangerous than those listed by Kaplan and Dorff. The increasing use of hydrogenated oils, and their linkage to heart disease, offers an additional area for concern. More than a billion pounds of hydrogenated oils are now used annually.

It is estimated that almost half of the American population, more than 100 million citizens, now suffer from some form of chronic illness, of which 25 million are allergic disorders. These allergies are increasingly found to be caused by exposure to or ingestion of some chemical substance. 20 million Americans have nervous disorders; 10 million have stomach ulcers; 700,000 suffer from cancer, and lesser numbers suffer from such diseases as lupus and muscular dystrophy.

In 1917-18, of the draftees for World War I, 21.3% were rejected and 9.9% placed in "limited service" because of various handicaps. In the Korean War period, after World War II, from 1947-1955, 52% of the draftees were rejected for physical and mental defects, a 21% increase since World War I, despite the great "advances" which the United States had supposedly made in nutrition, medical care, meals for school children, and other marks of progress. These figures also do not take into account that standards for World War I draftees were much higher than in World War II. In 1955, 25% of all draftees from New York City, aged from 21 to 26, were turned down for heart ailments. Of some 200 Americans killed in Korea, and autopsied, 80% were found to have advanced stages of heart disease. Dr. Jolliffe reported to Congress in 1955 that, "Whereas coronary heart disease was a rarity prior to 1920, it has now become the No. One cause of death in the 45 to 64 year old age group as well as after 65." How much of this was due to the increase in the use of chlorinated water supplies after World War I, Dr. Jolliffe does not say. Although specialists know that the ingestion of chlorine is a primary factor in the formation of arteriosclerotic plaques on the walls of arteries, no studies have been commissioned to determine the use of chlorine as a factor in the increase of deaths from heart failure. Dr.

Mendelsohn has noted, fluoridation of water is one of the Four Holy Waters of the Church of Modern Medicine. Scientists dare not tamper with what is essentially a religious and emotional conviction.

Dr. Mendelsohn also points out the possible contradictions in the American Medical Association's frequent admonitions to get your daily supply of the Big Four for adequate nutrition, that is, vegetables and fruits, grains, meats and dairy products. Dr. Mendelsohn points out that many groups cannot tolerate cow's milk because of enzymatic deficiencies. Some studies show that 75% of the world's peoples are lactose intolerant, and cannot digest cow's milk.

One of the post World War II epidemics was the worldwide reaction to the extensive use of DDT, even though DDT had come into being as the supposed guardian against epidemics during the war. Its use had been advertised as the miracle pesticide which would prevent outbreaks of various diseases in the war-ravaged nations of the world. However, DDT was eventually found to be a cumulative poison in the human system, much like sodium fluoride. Not only were considerable concentrations of DDT being accumulated in man's fatty tissues, but he also was consuming additional amounts in every forkful of food that he ate. Nobel Prize winner Dr. Otto Warburg heralded the dangers of DDT when he warned that any poison which interferes with the respiration of the cells causes irreparable damage and produces degenerative diseases such as cancer. Despite such warnings, from 1947 to 1956, the annual production of DDT quadrupled to an annual total of more than five hundred million pounds. The Public Health Service analyzed food in a Federal prison for DDT content, finding stewed fruit with 69 ppm content, bread with 100 ppm DDT content, while lard used in the preparation of food was estimated to have 2500 ppm DDT. Tests also showed that it took many years to lower the amount of DDT stored in body fat. DDT is even more persistent in soil; seven years after DDT was applied to test plots 80% of it remained. Orchards and farms which used DDT in annual spraying built up enormous amounts in the soil. DDT has since been banned, but the residues remain. Even after the ban, Monsanto continued to make huge profits from the sale of DDT by exporting it to other countries. Another commonly used pesticide, chloridane, was found to be four times as toxic as DDT. Another substance which was later banned was aramite, an acknowledged carcinogen used as a pesticide.

Produced by the chemical conglomerate, U.S. Rubber, in 1951, aramite came under a barrage of criticism. Despite the widespread publication of FDA tests proving its dangers, it remained in use until the spring of 1958, when it was finally withdrawn.

Some substances containing arsenic are still found in foodstuffs as pesticide residue and as a food additive for poultry and livestock. Selocide, a pesticide based on selenium, was found to produce cirrhosis of the liver in persons ingesting food which had been treated with this chemical. After two hundred children became ill from eating dyed popcorn at a Christmas party, the FDA announced decertification of the three dyes involved, Red No. 32, Orange 1 and Orange 2. A government report stated that,

"When FD&C Red No. 32 was fed to rats at a level of 2.0 per cent of the diet, all the rats died within a week. At a 1.0 per cent level, death occurred within 12 days. At 0.5 per cent, most of the rats died within 26 days. At 0.25 per cent approximately half of the rats died within 3 months. All of the rats showed marked growth retardation and anemia. Autopsy revealed moderate to marked liver damage. Similar but less severe results were obtained with rats on a diet containing 0.1 per cent of FD&C Red No. 32 ... Dogs taking 100 milligrams per kilogram of body weight per day showed moderate weight loss ... A single dose gave diarrhea in the majority of the dogs tested."

Tests of Orange No. 1 gave similar results as FD&C Red No. 32 More that half of the Florida orange crop was run through these dyes to give them a beautiful orange color, instead of the pale green which was their normal color at the time of picking. Canned and frozen orange juice often contained larger amounts of these dyes, because packers bought "packing house reject," which were deemed unsuitable for grocery store marketing.

Although the Christmas Party which highlighted the perils of these dyes took place in December 1955, manufacturers were told they could legally use up stocks of these colors. The ban went into effect February 15, 1956, but it had been in the making since December 19, 1953, two years before the near fatal party.

One of the more common food processes today is the hydrogenation process which destroys all nutritional value. The process consists of saturating the fatty acids with hydrogen under pressure, with temperatures up to 410 F. with a metal catalyst, either nickel, platinum or copper, for as long as eight hours; after this treatment, it becomes an inert or dead substance. Hydrogenated oils in margarine used for cooking break down into dangerous toxins when heated, although butter can be heated for long periods of time without forming toxins.

Despite the well publicized dangers of chemical food additives and other nutritional problems, the principal charitable health foundations have for years strongly opposed any linkage of diet, nutrition and health. This program was originally laid down for them many years ago by the famous quack, Morris Fishbein, and the American Medical Association. They have religiously followed these precepts, as coming from the original prophet, in the ensuing decades. AMA officials testified before a Senate Committee that there is no proof that diet is related to disease, adding the warning that changing American eating habits might lead to "economic dislocation." The Arthritis Foundation assures its place in the sun by regular reiterations of its claims that arthritis is incurable, although this has never prevented the foundation from annual fund-raising drives to collect money for a "cure." This foundation denounces any food supplements or health detoxification programs to cleanse the system, leaving this to the province of individualistic health care practitioners in California. The foundation also opposes the following of rotary diets which could uncover food allergies in arthritis patients. In 1985, the Arthritis Foundation collected $36.2 million, as one of a small group of "monopoly-disease" groups which have established their claim to a particular disease, a feature which is very attractive to the Medical Monopoly which approves their positions. Its sister foundations, National Multiple Sclerosis, United Cerebral Palsy, and the Lupus Foundation are equally protective towards their stakes in the "Monopoly diseases," which the Super Rich have staked out as well-defined and unchallengeable claims. Reports of cures of arthritis by abstaining from such acid- producing foods as beef, chocolate and milk, while routine, are totally denied by the Arthritis Foundation. One San Francisco doctor published his findings after curing the most advanced cases or rheumatoid arthritis by banning all fruits, meats, wheat and dairy products, a rigorous regimen which those patients willing to abide by it found to produce total relief.

The American Cancer Society also routinely branded all metabolic-nutritional approaches to cancer treatment as "anecdotal links to cancer prevention" which constitute "quackery," the famous designation for nonapproved medical treatment which was publicized for years by America's two most famous quacks, Simmons and Fishbein. However, in 1887, just after the founding of the New York Cancer hospital, an Albany, New York physician published a book, "Diet in Cancer," by Dr. Ephraim Cutter, Kellogg Books, pp. 19-26, in which he wrote, "Cancer is a disease of nutrition." In 1984, faced by a growing tide of publicity about the efficacy of diet and nutrition in many cancer cases, the American Cancer Society did a reluctant flipflop, offering the cautious assertion that diet and vitamins might offer some slight benefit. ACS continued to ignore the facts showing that the record of increase in the use of food additives paralleled the annual increase in the cancer toll. From 1940 to 1977, the American intake of food colorings and additives increased tenfold, while the per capita consumption of fruits and vegetables declined. Later studies have shown an inverse association between the daily intake of green or yellow vegetables and the mortality rates from cancer. Studies of victims of prostate cancer, now epidemic among American men, showed a high intake of fats, milk, meats and coffee. It was recommended that baked goods should be avoided, whether because of additives or the danger of aluminum compounds was not stated.

There has also been a fivefold increase in the intake of fried food in the United States, most of which has come through the "fast food" outlets. The use of fats in these outlets, with little supervision and inadequately trained personnel, means that deep frying fats are reused over long periods of time. These reused fats have been proved to be mutagenic in laboratory tests, and are listed as potentially carcinogenic by researchers.

The *Washington Post,* January 23, 1988, noted that of 60,000 chemicals now in general use, only two per cent have been tested for toxicity. Many Americans can testify about the drastic effects of many chemicals, especially pesticides.

Colman McCarthy recently complained in his *Washington Post* column that "The environmental war against bugs escalates as a war against people." The widespread use of such chemicals as sevin, malathion, and surban on private lawns, golf courses and public parks has resulted in a number of deaths, with an unknown number whose cause was never recorded. One man in a Washington suburb walked across a recently sprayed golf course; he went home and died. He had absorbed a lethal amount of pesticide through his lowcut ankle socks. A cardiovascular surgeon who has treated 17,000 patients in the last twelve years at his Environmental Health Center in Dallas estimates that between ten and twenty per cent of the American population is being seriously harmed by chemicals. Thousands of school children sit in classrooms for six hours a day breathing in residues of asbestos, formaldehyde and other chemicals, which the school officials have no idea are present.

One physician graphically recorded her illness in the *New Yorker*, January 4, 1988; she was suffering from a tightness in the chest, wheezing, gastro-intestinal problems, anorexia, nausea, vomiting and cramps, as well as weight loss, fatigue and general twitching. She sought aid from another physician, who was puzzled by these symptoms; she finally looked in a medical book, and found all of her symptoms listed together as the result of exposure to organophosphates pesticide. She had a weekend cottage in which her exterminator had used organophosphates to kill an invasion of small ants. On subsequent weekends, she had been sitting in the fumigation chamber whenever she went into her cottage; the exterminator had used Durshan, an organophosphate, and Ficam, a methyl carbonate. After finding out what her problem was, she was able to counter them with the recommended treatment, oral atropine, but she found that her system had now become sensitized to these pesticides. If she went into any area where they had been used, all of her symptoms returned.

This physician wryly pointed out that it is routine for physicians to diagnose her symptoms as psychosomatic, or even as mental illness; because she was a physician herself, the doctor she had consulted had not turned her away with this standard response, which is given with a prescription of liberal amounts of Valium or Librium. The list of poisons encountered in every day life is a long one. For years, people died suddenly from inhaling the fumes of a common cleaning agent, carbon tetrachloride, but it took years before it was finally withdrawn from general sale. Recent reports found that 35% of all chickens in grocery store meat boxes contain significant amounts of salmonella, a notorious cause of gastric illness and death.

Twelve million pounds of cyclamates a year are now used in foodstuffs; this is mostly produced by Abbott Laboratories. A University of Wisconsin study in 1966 recommended that cyclamates be removed from all foodstuffs. It was found that the ingestion of cyclamates affected the eye's reaction to light.

Cyclamates were also found to cause excess loss of potassium if a person was using one of the very common thiazide drugs for high blood pressure, as millions of Americans do. It was also found that cyclamates interfered with the action of diabetic drugs, although the purpose of the widespread use was advertised to be a solution to the problems of diabetics, who would thereby consume less sugar. It also shows indications of causing bladder cancer.

In Midland, Michigan, DOW Chemical had to shut down its 2,4,5T plant because the workers were suffering from Chloracne, a skin disease for which there is no known method of treatment. For years, oranges had been gussied up for public sale by coating them with biphenyl, the chemical which is used in the embalming process in mortuaries. One of the world's most widely consumed foodstuffs is pasta, the Italian word for paste. In fact, pasta, or spaghetti, is ground wheat which is mixed with water to form a paste. In libraries, it is known as library paste. Millions of people eat this congealed paste every day. Macaroni, another common food, is dehydrated concentrated starch. Milk is the most mucous-forming part of the average American diet; drinking milk causes the system to become clogged, resulting in colds, which often develop into flu, asthma or pneumonia. Some 75% of the world's population is unable to digest cow's milk, a fact which has never discouraged a single dairy company from advertising on television that "Milk Is Good For You."

Soft drinks contain large amounts of the chemical citric acid, which acts to increase the acidity level of the entire body. The results are frequently manifested as mouth cankers and duodenal ulcers. Caramel, also widely used, is prepared from ammonia; its ingestion causes mental disorders in children. Cola drinks, from a derivative of cocaine, increase heart action, cause irritability of the nerves and resultant insomnia, and can cause paralysis of the heart. Beer contains gypsum, which is better known as plaster of paris.

Hops in beer cause a hypnotic effect and can cause delirium tremens. (The only case of delirium tremens ever observed by the present writer occurred in a soldier who drank nothing stronger than beer. This puzzled me at the time, because I had always heard that delirium tremens was found only in those who ingested large quantities of hard liquor.)

Widely used food additives, colors and seasonings include cochineal, used to produce a bright red color; it is made from the bodies of dried lice. Food colors have been the subjects of warnings for many years; Arthur Kallet in 1933 published findings that the widely used colors Violet 1 and Citrus Red 2 (used for coloring oranges) were definitely carcinogenic. A few years ago, a number of health cure products featuring hexochlorophene, a highly recommended antiseptic substance, were hastily withdrawn from the market. It was found that phisohex, a product then used daily in every hospital in the United States, had caused death when rubbed on the skin of babies. Phisohex was also featured in feminine hygiene sprays, Dial soap, shampoos, toothpaste, and many feminine cosmetics; all of these products contained dangerous concentrations of hexachlorophene. Not only was it manufactured from the same chemical as DOW's deadly weedkillers, 2,4,5T and 2,4D; it is also closely related to the deadly dioxin, which has been much in the news. It was only after many years of health care use that products containing hexachlorophene were found to produce dangerous reactions in babies washed or rubbed with any products containing it, although the relationship with the deadly dioxin was only made public much later. Even with this revelation, it required a ten year struggle to get the highly profitable hexachlorophene products off the market.

The commonly used food colors amaranth (red); bordeaux (brown); orange (yellow); procean (scarlet) all are derived from compounding nitrogen and benzene (a distillate of coal), which is also a commonly used motor fuel. Manufacturers dye their beverages with napthol (yellow), guinea green, which is derived from the reaction of chloroform or benzene and aluminum chloride to produce a dark green; tartrazene (yellow) is manufactured by producing a reaction of acetophene on diazomethane to produce a poisonous chemical which is then used in coloring food.

Dr. Samuel West explains the death from shock, which often occurs just after an accident or an operation, results from trapped blood proteins, which attract excess sodium and cause the death of the body, beginning at the cell level.

Recommendations for better nutrition include eating starches with fats or green vegetables; eating fruits alone; and seasoning with herbs. The effect of herbs is that they work electrically on the system, meaning that they work quickly, and that they cause "miraculous" changes. The admonitions to drink cow's milk forbear from explaining that cow's milk is a substance far removed in nature from human mother's milk. It contains 300% more casein, because it is designed by nature for a calf which can increase its gross weight from one to two thousand pounds in six to eight weeks; no human grows at such a fast rate.

Alfalfa is a highly recommended substance by many nutritionists because of its structure; its chlorophyll molecule is a web of carbon and hydrogen, nitrogen and oxygen atoms grouped around a single atom of magnesium; this is similar to the structure of hemoglobin, the red corpuscle, except that the atoms are grouped around a single atom of iron instead of magnesium.

A recommended treatment for kidney stones is lemon juice in a glass of water, or a combination of carrot and beet juice. The present writer has obtained quick relief and shrinking of a kidney stone in the ureter by drinking quantities of cranberry juice. These juices apparently begin to dissolve the stone, which then passes without effort. The stone is usually an oxide, an accumulation of minerals or oxides which forms a hard stone.

Although canning of food became very popular during the nineteenth century, as an ideal method of preserving large quantities of food which would otherwise be thrown away, the canning process heats the food until it destroys the enzymes. Heating food over 130 degrees eliminates the enzymes, which are the keystone to growth in the system. Enzymes take on minerals and use them for growth.

The surplus of elements left over from the manufacture of atomic bombs now threatens us with another "magical" process, the process of preserving food by irradiating it. Cobalt 60, one of these atomic bomb leftovers, is now being offered to food irradiators for $100,000 per kilo. Should the food irradiation program fall through, this byproduct of atomic bombs will have to be disposed of by the manufacturer at great expense. It is a repetition of the dilemmas which brought us such public "boons" as chlorination of water after World War I and nitrate fertilizers after World War II.

The first commercial use of food irradiation took place in occupied West Germany in 1957, where it was used experimentally to sterilize spices used in the manufacture of sausages. The results were so disturbing that the West German government was forced to ban it in 1958. At the same time, the Soviet Union had begun to use irradiation to inhibit the sprouting of potatoes in storage; in 1959, the Soviets used it for the disinfestation of grain. Canada, which is heavily influenced by pro-Soviet representatives in its government, began to use irradiation on potatoes in 1960. The U.S. Food and Drug Cosmetic Act of 1958 took up the use of irradiation, defining it as an "additive," which brought it under their control. In 1963, the FDA gave permission for the use of irradiation to sterilize canned bacon; this permission was rescinded in 1968.

In 1968, the Rockefeller Monopoly moved to back the food irradiation process on a national level. The Coalition for Food Irradiation was formed by some of the nation's biggest food companies; ALPO, Beatrice, Campbell Soup,

Del Monte, Gaines Foods, General Foods, Hormel, Heinz, Hershey, Gerber, MARS, Stouffer and Welch. Joining them in the coalition were the chemical companies, W. R. Grace, DuPont and Rockwell International. The Coalition began the tried and true technique of staging well-planned and expensive "conferences" at prominent universities, at which only the advocates for their plan would be heard. One of these conferences backfired. The planned irradiation conference at Johns Hopkins University Center for Radiation Education and Research was scheduled in August 1987. Prospective attendees were disturbed to find that the list of scheduled speakers was heavily stacked in favor of food irradiation. Of the twenty listed speakers, nineteen were known proponents of irradiation. The sole critic of food irradiation, Rep. Douglas Bosco, of California, pulled out when he realized that he was being set up. It would be publicized that although critics of food irradiation had been given a place at the conference, the conclusions would be totally in favor of irradiation. The scheduled advocates of food irradiation included Dr. Ari Brynjolfsson of MIT; Dr. Ronald E. Engel, deputy administrator of the U.S. Dept. of Agriculture, which had approved the irradiation of pork; George Giddings, director of Isomedix, the nation's largest irradiation firm; Dennis Heldman, executive vice-president of National Food Processors, which planned a cesium irradiator with the Dept. of Agriculture in California; Dr. James H. Moy, a professor at the University of Hawaii, who proposed a cesium irradiator jointly with the Dept. of Agriculture in Hawaii. Johns Hopkins University was a willing participant in this staged conference because in 1986, it had received three hundred and seventeen million dollars in defense funds; Johns Hopkins University is the second largest defense contractor after MIT. Dr. Brynjolfsson of MIT was one of the earliest advocates of food irradiation.

The United States Army has spent some $50 million on food irradiation since the 1950s; most of the results have been flawed. Maine has outlawed the sale of irradiated food. Milwaukee forbade the building of an irradiation plant, and public opposition also forced Radiation Technology to abandon a plant in Elizabeth, New Jersey. In 1987, the European Parliament voted against irradiation in the European Community "on precautionary grounds." The Canadian parliament then decided against using irradiation for wheat. Meanwhile, Abbott Laboratories and Baxter Travenol, leading pharmaceutical manufacturers, have licensed Gamma Irradiation Facilities to DOW Corning, General Electric, General Foods, IBM, IRT Corporation, Merck, RCA and Rockwell International.

After the Canadian Parliament recommended against using irradiation for wheat, Hon. Jake Epp, Canadian Minister of Health and Welfare, announced that irradiation of the food supply would be permitted. This announcement, which Epp made on September 10, 1987, astounded many Canadians. It came after the recommendation against it of the Canadian Parliament, as well as after the condemnation of food irradiation by London's Food Commission in England. Here again, the desperation of the Chemical Trust leads it to imperil the health of a nation. There are many available records of tests indicating the dangers of irradiated foods. Consumption of irradiated rice has been linked with the development of pituitary, thyroid, heart and lung disturbances, and with the development of tumors. Children and test animals fed irradiated wheat developed increased polyphoidy (an abnormality of the chromosomes). In East/West magazine, Feb. 1988, a quote from an unclassified document from the Department of State on food irradiation, published in a congressional hearing on the pesticide Ethylene DiBromide, used on fruits and grains, is as follows:

"The Administration and Congress are interested in promoting the use of U.S. exclusive technology using cesium

137 isotope for the benefit of man. U.S. nuclear waste processing currently is producing the cesium isotope which Dept. of Energy would like to be used for beneficial purposes. Promulgation of cesium technology would benefit U.S. private sector activities and minimize U.S. nuclear waste disposal problems."

CHAPTER 9

THE DRUG TRUST

In 1987, the eighteen largest drug firms were ranked as follows:

1. Merck (U.S.) $4.2 billion in sales.
2. Glaxo Holdings (United Kingdom) $3.4 billion.
3. Hoffman LaRoche (Switzerland) $3.1 billion.
4. Smith Kline Beckman (U.S.) $2.8 billion.
5. Ciba-Geigy (Switzerland) $2.7 billion.
6. Pfizer (U.S.) $2.5 billion (Standard & Poor's gives its sales as $4 billion).
7. Hoechst A. G. (Germany) $2.5 billion (Standard & Poor's lists its sales as $38 billion Deutschmarks).
8. American Home Products (U.S.) $2.4 billion ($4.93 billion according to Standard & Poor's).
9. Lilly (U.S.) $2.3 billion ($3.72 billion Standard & Poor's).
10. Upjohn (U.S.) $2 billion.
11. Squibb (U.S.) $2 billion.
12. Johnson & Johnson (U.S.) $1.9 billion.
13. Sandoz (Switzerland) $1.8 billion.
14. Bristol Myers (U.S.) $1.6 billion.
15. Beecham Group (United Kingdom) $1.4 billion (Standard & Poor's gives $1.4 billion in sales of the U.S. subsidiary—$2.6 billion pounds sterling as overall income).

16. Bayer A. G. (Germany) $1.4 billion (Standard & Poor's gives the figure as $45.9 billion Deutschmarks).
17. Syntex (U.S.) $1.1 billion.
18. Warner Lambert (U.S.) $1.1 billion (Standard & Poor's gives the figure as $3.1 billion).

Thus we find that the United States still maintains an overwhelming lead in the production and sale of drugs. In the United States, the sale of prescription drugs rose in 1987 by 12.5% to $27 billion. Eleven of the eighteen leading firms are located in the United States; three in Switzerland; two in Germany; and two in the United Kingdom. Nutritionist T. J. Frye notes that the Drug Trust in the United States is controlled by the Rockefeller group in a cartel relationship with I. G. Farben of Germany. In fact, I. G. Farben was the largest chemical concern in Germany during the 1930s, when it engaged in an active cartel agreement with Standard Oil of New Jersey. The Allied Military Government split it up into three companies after World War II, as part of the "anti-cartel" goals of that period, which was not unlike the famed splitting up of Standard Oil itself by court order, while the Rockefellers maintained controlling interest in each of the new companies. In Germany, General William Draper, of Dillon Read investment bankers, unveiled the new decree from his office in the I. G. Farben building. Henceforth, I. G. Farben would exist no more; instead, three companies would emerge—Bayer, of Leverkusen; BASF at Ludwigshafen; and Hoescht, near Frankfort. Each of the three spawns is now larger than the old I. G. Farben; only ICI of England is larger. These firms export more than half of their product. BASF is represented in the United States by Shearman and Sterling, the Rockefeller law firm of which William Rockefeller is a partner.

The world's No. 1 drug firm, Merck, began as an apothecary shop in Darmstadt, Germany, in 1668. Its president, John J. Horan, is a partner of J. P. Morgan Company, and the Morgan Guaranty Trust. He attended a Bilderberger meeting in Rye, New York, May 10-12, 1985. In 1953, Merck absorbed another large drug firm, Sharp & Dohme. At that time, Oscar Ewing, the central figure in the government fluoridation promotion for the Aluminum Trust, was secretary of the Merck firm, his office then being at One Wall Street, New York.

Directors of Merck include John T. Connor, who began his business career with Cravath, Swaine and Moore, the law firm for Kuhn, Loeb Company; Connor then joined the Office of Naval Research, became Special Assistant to the Secretary of the Navy 1945-47, became president of Merck, then president of Allied Stores from 1967-80, then chairman of Schroders, the London banking firm. Connor is also a director of a competing drug firm, Warner Lambert, director of the media conglomerate Capital Cities ABC, and director of Rockefeller's Chase Manhattan Bank. Each of the major drug firms in the United States has at least one director with close Rockefeller connections, or with a Rothschild bank. Another director of Merck is John K. McKinley, chief operating officer of Texaco; he is also a director of Manufacturers Hanover Bank, which Congressional records identify as a major Rothschild bank.

McKinley is also a director of the aircraft firm, Martin Marietta, Burlington Industries, and is a director of the aircraft firm, Martin Marietta, Burlington Industries, and is a director of the Rockefeller- controlled Sloan Kettering Cancer Institute. Another Merck director is Ruben F. Mettler, chairman of the defense contractor TRW, Inc.; he was formerly chief of the Guided Missiles Department at Ramo- Wooldridge, and has received the human relations award from the National Conference of Christians and Jews—he is also a director of Bank of America.

Other directors of Merck include Frank T. Cary, who was chairman of IBM for many years; he is also a director of Capital Cities ABC, and partner of J. P. Morgan Company; Lloyd C. Elam, president of Meharry Medical College, Nashville, TN, the nation's only black medical college. Elam is also a director of the American Psychiatric Association, Nashville City Bank, and the Alfred P. Sloan Foundation, which gives him a close connection to Rockefeller's Sloan Kettering Cancer Center; Marian Sulzberger Heiskell, heiress of the New York Times fortune. She was married to Orville Dryfoos, the paper's editor, who died of a heart attack during a newspaper strike; she then married Andrew Heiskell in a media merger—he was chairman of *Time* magazine and had been with the Luce organization for fifty years. She is also a director of Ford Motor. Heiskell is director of People for the American Way, a political activist group, chairman of the New York Public Library, and the Book-of-the-Month Club. Also on the board of Merck is a family member, Albert W. Merck; Reginald H. Jones, born in England, formerly chairman of General Electric, now chairman of the Board of Overseers, Wharton School of Commerce, director of Allied Stores and General Signal Corporation; Paul G. Rogers, who served in Congress from the 84th to the 95th Congresses; he was chairman of the important subcommittee on health; in 1979, he joined the influential Washington law firm and lobbyist, Hogan and Hartson. He is also a director of the American Cancer Society, the Rand Corporation, and Mutual Life Insurance.

Thus we find that the world's No. 1 drug firm has two directors who are partners of J. P. Morgan Company, one who is director of Rockefeller's Chase Manhattan Bank and one who is director of the Rothschild Bank, Manufacturers Hanover; most of the directors are connected with vital defense industries, and interlock with other defense firms. On the board of TRW, of which Ruben Mettler is chairman, is William H. Krome George, former chairman of ALCOA, and Martin Feldstein, former economic advisor to President Reagan. The major banks, defense firms, and prominent political figures interlock with the CIA and the drug firms.

The No. 2 drug firm is Glaxo Holdings, with $3.4 billion in sales. Its chairman is Austin Bide; deputy chairman is P. Girolami, who is a director of National Westminster Bank, one of England's Big Five. Directors are Sir Alistair Frame, chairman of Rio Tinto Zinc, one of the three firms which are the basis of the Rothschild fortune; Frame is also on the board of another Rothschild holding, the well known munitions firm, Vickers; also Plessey, another defense firm which recently bid on a large contract with the U.S. Army; Frame is president of Britoil, and director of Glaxo are Lord Fraser of Kilmarnock, who was deputy chairman of the Conservative Party (now the ruling party in England) from 1946 to 1975, when he joined Glaxo; Lord Fraser was also a member of the influential Shadow cabinet; B. D. Taylor, counselor of Victoria College of Pharmacy and chairman of Wexham Hospital; J. M. Raisman, chairman of Shell Oil UK Ltd., another Rothschild controlled firm. Lloyd's Bank, one of the Big Five, British Telecommunications, and the Royal Committee on Environmental Pollution; Sir Ronald Arculus, retired from Her Majesty's Diplomatic Service after a distinguished career; he had served in San Francisco, New York, Washington and Paris; he was then appointed Ambassador to Italy, and was the UK Delegate to the United Nations Convention on the Law of the Sea, which sought to apportion marine wealth among the have-not countries: Arculus is now a director of Trusthouse Forte Hotels, and London and Continental Bankers; and Professor R. G. Dahrendorf, one of the world's most active sociologists and a longtime Marxist propagandist. Dahrendorf, a director of the Ford Foundation since 1976, is a graduate of the London School of Economics, professor of sociology at Hamburg and Tubingen, parliamentary Secretary of State at the Foreign Office, West Germany since 1969, and has received honors from Senegal, Luxemburg and Leopold II.

The Rothschilds apparently appointed Dahrendorf a director of Glaxo because of his emphatic Marxist pronunciamentos. The European director of the Ford Foundation, he claims, in his book, "Marx in Perspective," that Marx is the greatest factor in the emergence of modern society. Dahrendorf's principal contribution to sociology has been his well-advertised concept of the "new man," whom he has dubbed "homo sociologicus," a being who has been transformed by socialism into a person whose every disctinctive feature, including racial characteristics, have disappeared. He is the modern robot, a uniform creature who can easily be controlled by the force of world socialism. Dahrendorf is the apostle of the modern faith that there are no racial differences in any of the various races of mankind; he denounces any mention of "superiority" or of differing skills as "ideological distortion." Dahrendorf is a prominent member of the Bilderbergers; he attended their meeting at Rye, New York from May 10-12, 1985. He is professor of Sociology at Konstanz University, as well as his other previously mentioned posts.

Thus we find that the world's No. 2 drug firm is directed by two of the Rothschild's family's most trusted henchmen and by the world's most outspoken explicator of Marxism.

The world's No. 3 drug firm, Hoffman LaRoche of Switzerland, is still controlled by members of the Hoffman family, although there have been rumors of takeover attempts in recent years. The firm was founded by Fritz Hoffman, who died in 1920. The firm's first big seller was Siropin in 1896; its sales of Valium and Librium now amount to one billion dollars a year; its subsidiary spread the dangerous chemical, dioxin, over the Italian town, Seveso, which cost $150 million to clean up in a 10 year campaign.

His son's widow, Maya Sacher, is now married to Paul Sacher, a musician who is conductor of the Basle Chamber Orchestra. Hoffman had added his wife's name, LaRoche, to the family company, as is the custom in Europe; the Hoffmans still control 75% of the voting shares. The Sachers have one of the world's most expensive art collections, Old Masters and modern paintings.

In 1987, Hoffman LaRoche tried to take over Sterling Drug, a venture in which they were aided by Lewis Preston, chairman of J. P. Morgan Company; he also happened to be Sterling's banker. In the ensuing brouha-ha, Preston decided to retire. Eastman Kodak then bought Sterling, with backing from the Rockefellers. The chairman of Hoffman LaRoche is Fritz Gerber, a 58 year old Swiss army colonel. The son of a carpenter, he became a lawyer, then chairman of Hoffman LaRoche. Gerber is also a director of Zurich Insurance; thus he is associated with Switzerland's two biggest firms; he draws a salary of 2.3 million Swiss francs per year, plus a $1.7 million working agreement with Glaxo holdings.

Hoffman LaRoche received a great deal of publicity in April 1988 because of unfavorable revelations about its acne drug, "Accutane" after the Food and Drug Administration publicized figures that the drug had caused 1000 spontaneous abortions, 7000 other abortions, and other side effects such as joint aches, drying of skin and mucous membranes, and hair loss. Hoffman LaRoche was faulted by FDA for purposely omitting women, and particularly pregnant women, from the studies on which it based requests for approval of Accutane. The company was aware that Accutane caused serious effects when taken during pregnancy.

Hard on the heels of the Accutane revelations, Hoffman LaRoche made new headlines in the Wall Street Journal with Congressman Ted Weiss's demand, reported on May 6,

1988, that a criminal investigation be launched of the forty deaths, recorded since 1986, caused by taking Versed, Hoffman La-Roche's tranquilizer which is a chemical cousin of its best selling drug, Valium.

The No. 4 drug firm, Smith Kline Beckman, banks with the Mellon Bank. Its chairman, Robert F. Dee, is a director of General Foods, Air Products and Chemical and the defense firm, United Technologies, which interlocks with Citibank. Directors are Samuel H. Ballam, Jr., chairman of the Hospital of the University of Pennsylvania, director of American Water-Works, Westmoreland Coal Company, General Coal Company, INA Investment Securities, chairman of CIGNA's High Yield Fund, and Geothermal Resources International; Francis P. Lucier, chairman of Black & Decker; Donald P. McHenry, former U.S. Ambassador to the UN, 1979-81, now international advisor to the Council on Foreign Relations, Trustee of Brookings Institution and the Carnegie Endowment for International Peace, Ford Foundation, and the super-secret Ditchley Foundation set up by W. Averell Harriman during World War II; McHenry is also a director of Coca Cola and International Paper; Carolyn K. Davis, who was dean of the school of nurses at University of Michigan 1973-75, Health and Human Services since 1981; she is also a director of Johns Hopkins.

Other directors of Smith Kline are Andrew L. Lewis, Jr., chairman of Union Pacific, the basis of the Harriman fortune; he is director of Ford Motor, trustee in bankruptcy Reading Company, former chairman of Reagan's transition team and deputy director of the Republican National Committee; R. Gordon McGovern, chairman of Campbell Soup; Ralph A. Pfeiffer, Jr., chairman of IBM World Trade Corporation, American International Far East Corporation, Riggs National Bank, and chairman U.S.-China Trade Commission; he is also vice chairman of the key foreign policy operation, Center for Strategic and International Studies, which was founded by Jeane Kirkpatrick's husband, Evron Kirkpatrick of the CIA.

The world's No. 5 drug firm, Ciba-Geigy of Switzerland, does a billion dollar a year business in the United States, and operates ten drug factories here.

Pfizer, No. 6 in size of the world's drug firms, does $4 billion a year, according to Standard & Poor's; the company banks with Rockefeller's Chase Manhattan Bank. Pfizer's chairman, Edmund T. Pratt, Jr., was controller of IBM from 1949 to 1962; he is now a director of Chase Manhattan Bank, General Motors, International Paper, the Business Council and the Business Roundtable, two Establishment organizations; he is also chairman of the Emergency Committee for American Trade. Pfizer's president is Gerald Laubach, who joined Pfizer in 1950; he is a member of the council of Rockefeller University, and director of CIGNA, Loctite, and General Insurance Corporation; Barber Conable is director of Pfizer; he was a Congressman representing New York from 1965 to 1985, which would indicate a close Rockefeller connection; Conable is now president of the World Bank. Other directors of Pfizer are Joseph B. Flavin, chief operating officer of the 2½ billion a year Singer Company. Flavin was with IBM World Trade Corporation from 1953-1967, then president of Xerox; he is now with the Committee for Economic Development, Stamford Hospital, Cancer Research Foundation, and the National Council of Christians and Jews; Howard C. Kauffman, has been president of EXXON since 1975; he was previously regional coordinator in Latin America for EXXON, then president of Esso Europe in London; he is also a director of Celanese and Chase Manhattan Bank; his office is at One Rockefeller Plaza; James T. Lynn, who was general counsel for the U.S. Department of Commerce from 1969-71, then Under Secretary of State 1971-73, and then secretary of

HUD 1973-75, succeeding George Romney in that post; Lynn was editor of the *Harvard Law Review,* then joined Jones, Day, Reavis and Pogue in 1960 (a large Washington lobbying firm); Lynn accompanied Peter Peterson, then Secretary of Commerce, formerly chairman of Kuhn, Loeb Company, to Moscow in 1972, to conclude a trade agreement with the Soviets; this agreement was concluded in October, 1972; John R. Opel, president of IBM, director of the Federal Reserve Bank of New York, Time and the Institute for Advanced Study; Walter B. Wriston, chairman of Citicorp, director of General Electric, Chubb, New York Hospital, Rand Corporation and J. C. Penney.

Other directors of Pfizer are Grace J. Fippinger, secretary- treasurer of the $10 billion a year NYNEX Corporation; she is an adviser to Manufacturers Hanover, the Rothschild Bank, director of Bear Stearns investment bankers, Gulf & Western Corporation, Connecticut Mutual Life Insurance and honorary member of the board of the American Cancer Society; Stanley O. Ikenberry, president of the University of Illinois, director of Harris Bankcorp, Carneigie Foundation for the Advancement of Teaching; William J. Kennedy, chief operating officer of North Carolina Mutual Life, director of Quaker Oats (with Frank Carlucci, who is now Secretary of Defense), Mobil (with Alan Greenspan, who is now Chairman of the Federal Reserve System Board of Governors—Greenspan was a delegate to the Bilderberger meeting in Rye, New York, May 10-12, 1985); Paul A. Marks, chief of Sloan Kettering Cancer Center since 1980; he is a biologist, professor of human genetics at Cornell, and adjunct professor at Rockefeller University, visiting professor at Rockefeller University Hospital; he is also with National Institute of Health, Dreyfus Mutual Fund, director of cancer treatment at the National Cancer Institute, director of American Association for Cancer Research, served on the President's Cancer Panel from 1976 to 1979, and the Presidential Commission on the

Accident at Three Mile Island; he is a director of the $100 million Revson Foundation (cosmetics fortune), with Simon Rifkind and Benjamin Buttenweiser, whose wife was attorney for Alger Hiss while Buttenweiser was Assistant High Commissioner for occupied West Germany.

Of the major drug firms, none shows more direct connections with the Rockefeller interests than Pfizer, which banks with the Rockefeller bank, Chase Manhattan, has as director Howard Kaufmann, president of Exxon, and Paul Marks of the Rockefeller controlled Sloan Kettering Cancer Center and Rockefeller Hospital. In most cases, only one Rockefeller connection is needed to assure control of a corporation.

The No. 7 in world ranked drug firms is Hoechst A. G. of Germany, a spinoff from I. G. Farben, i.e., Rockefeller Warburg Rothschild control. It operates a number of plants in the U.S., including American Hoechst at Somerville, New Jersey, and Hoechst Fibers Company. Hoechst manufactures the widely used polyester fiber Trevira, antibiotic food additives for swine and broilers (Flavomycin), and other pharmaceuticals used in animal raising.

No. 8 in world ranking, American Home Products banks at the Rothschild Bank, Manufacturers Hanover, and does $3.8 billion a year ($4.93 according to Standard & Poor's). It became even larger by its recent purchase of A. H. Robins Drug Company of Richmond, VA. A. H. Robins had gone into bankruptcy after facing $2.5 billion in payments to some 200,000 women who had been injured by its Dalkon Shield, an intrauterine device. An inadequately tested vagina clamp caused severe damage to many women. A French firm, Sanofi, then attempted to buy the firm, but was beaten out when American Home decided to pay a premium price for the firm's well known brand names, Chapstick and Robitussin. American Home's CEO is John W. Culligan, who has been with the firm since 1937; he is a Knight of Malta, director of Mellon Bank, Carnegie Mellon University, American Standard, and Valley Hospital; president of American Home is John R. Stafford, director of the Rothschild Bank, Manufacturers Hanover; he was formerly general counsel for the No. 3 ranked drug firm, Hoffmann LaRoche, and partner of the influential law firm, Steptoe and Johnson. Directors are K. R. Bergethon of Norway, now president of Lafayette College; A. Richard Diebold; Paul R. Frohring, and head of the Pharmaceutical Division of the War Production Board from 1942 to 1946; he is now trustee of John Cabot College, Rome, overseer of Case Western Reserve University, Mercy Hospital, Navy League, and the Biscayne Yacht Club; William F. LaPorte, who is director of Manufacturers Hanover Trust, American Standard, B. F. Goodrich, Dime Savings Bank, and president of the Buck Hill Falls Company; John F. McGillicuddy, chairman of Manufacturers Hanover Bank, who recently replaced Lewis Preston of J. P. Morgan Company as director of the Federal Reserve Bank of New York (Preston had been criticized for his role in promoting a deal for Hoffman LaRoche while engaged as Sterling Drug's banker); John F. Torell III, president of the Manufacturers Hanover Trust and Manufacturers Hanover Corporation; H. W. Blades, who was formerly president of Wyeth Labs, and is now director of Provident Mutual Life Insurance, Wistar International, Philadelphia National Bank, and Bryn Mawr Hospital; Robin Chandler Duke, of the tobacco family; Edwin A. Gee, director of Air Products and Chemical, International Paper, Bell & Howell; he is now chairman of International Paper and Canadian International Paper; Robert W. Sarnoff, son of David Sarnoff, who founded the RCA empire; and William Wrigley, chairman of the Wrigley Corporation, director of Texaco and the Boulevard National Bank of Chicago.

No. 9 in world ranking is Eli Lilly Company, whose chairman Richard D. Wood is also director of Standard Oil of Indiana, Chemical Bank New York, Elizabeth Arden, IVAC Corporation, Cardiac Pacemakers Inc., Elanco Products, Dow Jones, Lilly Endowment, Physio-Control Corporation, and the American Enterprise Institute for Public Policy Research, a supposedly rightwing thinktank in Washington where Jeane Kirkpatrick reigns supreme. Directors of Lilly are Steven C. Beering, born in Berlin, Germany, now president of Purdue University; he serves on numerous medical boards, Diabetes Association, Endocrine Association and is a director of Arvin Industries; Randall H. Tobias, is a director of the Bretton Woods Committee, has been with Bell Telephone Labs since 1964, now director of AT&T and Home Insurance Corporation; Robert C. Seamans, Jr. who was Secretary of the Air Force from 1969-1973, now director of the Carnegie Institute, Smithsonian Museum and National Geographic Society (with Laurance Rockefeller); He is also a director of Combustion Engineering, a firm which is engaged in a number of deals with the Soviet Union, Putnams Funds, a New England powerhouse investment firm; other directors of Lilly are J. Clayton LaForce, a Fulbright scholar, now director of the Rockefeller-funded National Bureau for Economic Research, and is dean of the graduate school of management at the University of California. LaForce is an influential member of the secretive Mont Pelerin Society, which represents the Viennese school of economics, a Rothschild sponsored enterprise which features Milton Friedman as its mouthpiece—it is actually a pseudo-rightwing think-tank run by William Buckley and the CIA. LaForce is also a trustee of the pseudo rightwing thinktank, Hoover Institution of Stanford University, which is run by two directors of the Rockefeller-funded League for Industrial Democracy, the leading Trotskyite thinktank, Sidney Hook and Seymour Martin Lipset. Other directors of Lilly are J. Paul Lyet II, chairman of the giant defense firm Sperry Corporation—two-thirds of its contracts are with government agencies; Lyet is also a director of Eastman Kodak, which has just purchased Sterling Drug; he is also a director of Armstrong World Industries, NL Industries and the Continental Group; Alva Otis Way III, president of American Express, director of Schroder Bank and Trust, formerly chairman—also director of Shearson Lehman, which now incorporates Kuhn, Loeb Company and Lehman Brothers, director of Firemans Fund Insurance Company and American International Banking Corporation, Warnex Ampex Communications Corporation; C. William Verity, Jr., whose father founded Armco Steel; a Yale graduate, Verity is now chairman of Armco; he was recently appointed Secretary of Commerce to replace fellow Yale man Malcolm Baldrige, a director of the defense firm Scovill Manufacturing—Baldrige had fallen off of a horse.

Verity is also a director of Chase Manhattan Bank, Mead Corporation and Taft Broadcasting. Verity was chosen as Secretary of Commerce because of his longtime record of agitation on behalf of the super-secret group, the U.S.-U.S.S.R. Trade & Economic Council, also known as USTEC, whose records are classified as Top Secret—several lawsuits are now under way to force the government to release USTEC documents under the Freedom of Information Act, but so far government attorneys have fought off all attempts to find out what this group is doing. Supposedly a cordial group of well-meaning American businessmen meeting with their smiling Soviet counterparts, USTEC was the brainchild of a top KGB official, who promoted it at the 1973 summit meeting between President Nixon and Brezhnev. The go-between was Donald Kendall of Pepsicola, who had just concluded a major trade deal with Russia; part of the price was Kendall's selling USTEC to the White House Team. Without Kendall, USTEC might never have gotten off the ground. The real goal of USTEC was voiced by H. Rowan Gaither, head of the Ford Foundation, when he was interviewed by foundation investigator, Norman Dodd. Gaither complained about the bad press the

Ford Foundation was receiving, claiming it was unjustified. "Most of us here," he exclaimed in self- exculpation, "were at one time or another, active in either the OSS or the State Department, or the European Economic Administration. During those times, and without exception, we operated under directives issued from the White House, the substance of which was to the effect that we should make every effort to alter life in the United States so as to make possible a comfortable merger with the Soviet Union."

USTEC is an important step in the merger program. Alva Way, president of American Express, serves on the board of Eli Lilly with C. William Verity. Way's fellow executive, James D. Robinson III, who is chairman of American Express, is a prime mover in USTEC, as is Robert Roosa, partner in Brown Brothers Harriman investment banking firm, who is executive officer of the Trilateral Commission. Other important USTEC members are Edgar Bronfman, head of the World Zionist Congress, chairman of Seagrams, the Bronfman family firm, and controlling a sizeable part of DuPont's stock, 21%; Maurice Greenberg, chairman of American International Group; Dr. Armand Hammer, longtime friend of the Soviet Union, and Dwayne Andreas, grain tycoon who is head of Archer-Daniels-Midland Corporation. Andreas, who financed CREEP, the organization which brought about the resignation of Richard Nixon from the presidency of the United States, has on his board Robert Strauss, former chairman of the Democratic National Committee, and Mrs. Nelson Rockefeller.

In 1972, a meeting was called in Washington at the ultra-exclusive F. Street Club, which had long been the secret meeting place for the top wheelers and dealers in Washington. Donald Kendall had invited David Rockefeller, who had opened a branch of Chase Manhattan in Red Square, Moscow, Helmut Sonnenfeldt of the State Department, who reputedly had been Henry Kissinger's "control" when Kissinger came to the United States as a double agent under Sonnenfeldt's patronage, and Georgi Arbatov, the well known Soviet propagandist in the United States. Arbatov told the group who Soviet Russia wanted on the board of the prospective organization, which became USTEC. He wanted Dr. Armand Hammer, Reginald Jones of General Electric, Frank Cary of IBM, and Irving Shapiro, head of DuPont. USTEC's ostensible purpose was to promote trade between the U.S. and Russia; its real purpose was to rescue the floundering Soviet economy and save its leaders from a disastrous revolution. The U.S. offered high technology, grain and military goods; the Russians offered to continue the Communist system.

The world's tenth largest drug firm is Upjohn, which is heavily into the production of agricultural chemicals such as Asgrow.

Upjohn has now been taken over by the leading defense firm, Todd Shipyards, whose directors include Harold Eckman, a director of W. R. Grace, the Bank of New York, Centennial Life Insurance Company, Home Life Insurance Company—he is the chairman of Atlantic Mutual Insurance Company, and Union de Seguros of Mexico: Raymond V. O'Brien, Jr., chairman of Emigrant Savings Bank of New York, and the International Shipholding Corporation; R. T. Parfet, Jr., who is chairman of Upjohn, director of Michigan Bell Telephone; Lawrence C. Hoff, who is chairman of the National Foundation for Infectious Diseases, and the American Foundation for Pharmaceutical Education; he is on the board of Sloan Kettering Cancer Institute, and was Under Secretary of Health at HEW from 1974-77; he is director of the National Heart & Lung Institute, and the U.S. Public Health Service Pharmacy Board; P. H. Bullen, who was with IBM from 1946-71, now operates as Bullen Management Company; Donald F. Hornig, professor and director of the Interdisciplinary Progress in Health at the

Harvard University School of Public Health; he is a director of Westinghouse Electric, and was group leader at Los Alamos in the development of the atomic bomb; he was special adviser in science at the U.S. Public Health Service from 1964 to 1969; he has received Guggenheim and Fullbright fellowships; Preston S. Parish, chairman of the executive committee at Upjohn, is a trustee of Williams College, Bronson Methodist Hospital, chairman of trustees for the W. E. Upjohn Unemployment Corporation, chairman of Kal-Aero, American National Holding Company and co-chairman of the Food and Drug Law Institute; William D. Mulholland, chairman of the Bank of Montreal, in which the Bronfmans have controlling interest— Charles Bronfman is a director. Mulholland is also a director of Standard Life Assurance Company of Edinburgh, Scotland, a director of Kimberly-Clark, Canadian Pacific Railroad, Harris Bancorp, and the Bahamas and Caribbean Ltd. branch of the Bank of Montreal. Mulholland was a general partner of Morgan Stanley from 1952 to 1969, when he became president of Brinco, a Rothschild holding company in Canada from 1970 to 1974.

Mulholland is also a director of Allgemeine Credit Anstalt of Frankfort (birthplace of the Rothschild family). Also director of Upjohn is William N. Hubbard, Jr., a director of Johnson Controls, Consumers Power Company a 3½ billion a year operation, formerly president of Upjohn, and dean of the medical college at New York University.

The 11th largest drug firm, E. E. Squibb, has as chairman Richard E. Furlaud; he is a director of the leading munitions firm Olin Corporation, and was general counsel for Olin from 1957- 1966. Furlaud was an attorney with the prominent Wall Street law firm, Root, Ballantine, Harlan, Busby and Palmer, founded by Elihu Root, Wilson's Secretary of State, who rushed $100 million from Wilson's personal War Fund to Soviet Russia to save the tottering

Bolshevik regime in 1917. Furlaud is a trustee of Rockefeller University and the Sloan Kettering Cancer Institute, which shows a Rockefeller connection at Squibb. Directors of Squibb include J Richardson Dilworth, the longtime financial trustee for all the members of the Rockefeller family. Dilworth married into the wealthy Cushing family, and was a partner of Kuhn, Loeb Company from 1946 to 1958, when his partner, Lewis Strauss of Kuhn, Loeb, retired as financial advisor to the Rockefellers. Dilworth took the job full time in 1958, taking over the entire 56th floor of Rockefeller Center, where he handled every bill incurred by any member of the family unit 1981. He is now chairman of the board of Rockefeller Center, director of Nelson Rockefeller's International Basic Economy Corporation, Chrysler, R. H. Macy, Colonial Williamsburg (another Rockefeller family enterprise), and Rockefeller University. He is trustee of the Yale Corporation and of the Metropolitan Museum, and director of Selected Investments of Luxemburg. Other directors of Squibb are Louis V. Gerstner, president of American Express, director of Caterpillar Tractor and longtime board member of Sloan Kettering Cancer Institute; Charles G. Koch, head of the family firm, Koch Enterprises, a $3 billion a year operation in Kansas City. Koch has a $500 million fortune, and personally bankrolled the supposedly rightwing organizations, the Cato Institute, the Mr. Pelerin Society, and the Libertarian Party. Koch Industries banks solely with Morgan Guaranty Trust, which brings it into the orbit of the J. P. Morgan Company.

Other directors of Squibb are Helen M. Ranney, chairman of the department of medicine of the University of California at San Diego since 1973; she was with Presbyterian Hospital New York from 1960 to 1964, and is a member of the American Society of Hematology; Robert W. van Fossan, chairman of Mutual Benefit Life Insurance, director of Long Island Public Service Gas & Electric,

Amerada Hess and Nova Pharmaceutical Corporation; Sanford H. McDonnell, chairman of the defense firm, McDonnell Douglas Aircraft Corporation; he is a director of Centerre Bancorp and the Navy League; Robert H. Ebert, dean of the medical school at Harvard since 1964; he is a trustee of the Rockefeller Foundation, the Population Council and president of the influential Milbank Memorial Fund, director of the Robert W. Johnson Foundation from the Johnson & Johnson pharmaceutical fortune; Ebert was a Rhodes Scholar and a Markle Scholar; Burton E. Sobel, director of the cardiac division at Washington University since 1973, National Institute of Health, editor of *Clinical Cardiology, American Journal of Cardiology, American Journal of Physiology* and many other medical positions; Rawleigh Warner, Jr., chairman of the giant Mobil Corporation, and director of many companies including AT&T, Allied Signal (the $9 billion a year defense firm), American Express, Chemical Bank, (also on the board of Signal was John F. Connally, former Secretary of the Treasury, and Carla Hills, former Secretary of HUD, whose husband was chairman of the Securities and Exchange Commission); Eugene F. Williams, director of the defense firm Olin Corporation and Emerson Electric. Squibb recently established a research institute at Oxford University with a $20 million donation; it also maintains the Squibb Institute for Medical Research in the United States. The scion of the family is Senator Lowell Weicker, a liberal who consistently votes against the Republican Party, of which he is a member. He is shielded from party discipline by his family fortune.

Twelfth in ranking of the world's drug firms is Johnson & Johnson; its chairman James E. Burke, is also a director of IBM and Prudential Insurance. President of Johnson & Johnson is David R. Clare; he is on the board of MIT and is a director of Motorola and of Overlook Hospital. Directors are William O. Baker, research chemist at Bell Tel labs from 1939 to 1980. A specialist in polymer research, Baker is on the boards of many organizations, and serves on the President's Intelligence Advisory Board. He is a consultant to the National Security Agency, consultant to the Department of Defense since 1959, trustee of Rockefeller University, General Motors, Cancer Research Foundation and the Robert A. Welch Foundation; Thomas S. Murphy, chairman of the media conglomerate, Capital Cities ABC, director of Texaco; Clifton E. Garvin, chairman of Exxon since 1947, the capstone of the Rockefeller fortune; he is also a director of Citicorp and Citibank, TRW, the defense firm, J. C. Penney, Pepsi Cola, Sperry, vice chairman of the Sloan Kettering Cancer Center, chairman of the Business Roundtable, and trustee of the Teachers Annuity Association of America.

Also director of Johnson & Johnson is Irving M. London, chairman of the Albert Einstein College of Medicine since 1970, professor of medicine at Harvard and MIT, Rockefeller Fellow in medicine at Columbia University, consultant to the Surgeon General of the United States; Paul J. Rizzo, vice chairman of IBM, and the Morgan Stanley Group; Joan Ganz Cooney, who is married to Peter Peterson, the former chairman of Kuhn, Loeb Company. She is president of Children's TV Workshop, director of the Chase Manhattan Bank, the Chase Manhattan Group, May Department stores and Xerox. She had been a publicist for NBC since 1954, when she developed her profitable children's television program.

She received the Stephen S. Wise award.

Number thirteen in world ranking is Sandoz of Switzerland.

Lysergic acid, the famous LSD, was developed in Sandoz laboratories in 1943 by chemist Dr. Albert Hofmann. Sandoz has $5 billion a year in business revenues including

$500 million in agricultural chemicals and dyestuffs produced by its American factories. Sandoz owns Northrup King, the huge hybrid seed company, Viking Brass and other firms.

Fourteenth in world ranking is Bristol Myers. Its chief operating officer is Richard Gelb, formerly with Clairol, the company which had been founded by his family. Gelb is chairman of the Rockefeller controlled Sloan Kettering Cancer Center; he is a director of the Federal Reserve Bank of New York, Cluett Peabody, New York Times, New York Life Insurance, Bankers Trust, the Council of Foreign Relations, the Business Council and the Business Roundtable. Directors of Bristol-Myers include Ray C. Adam, a partner of J. P. Morgan Company and director of Morgan Guaranty Trust, Metropolitan Life, Cities Service, and chairman of the $2 billion a year NL Industries, a petroleum field service concern; William M. Ellinghaus, who has been with the Bell Systems since 1940, president of New York Telephone, director of J. C. Penney, Bankers Trust, vice chairman of the New York Stock Exchange, International Paper, Armstrong World Industries, New York Blood Center and United Way; he is a Knight of Malta of the Holy Sepulcher of Jerusalem, president of AT&T, director of Textron, Revlon and Pacific Tel & Tel; John D. Macomber, chairman of Celanese, director of the Chase Manhattan Bank, RJR Industries, Nabisco; Martha R. Wallace, member of the Trilateral Commission, management consultant to Department of State from 1951-53, now director of RCA, *Fortune, Time,* Henry Luce Foundation and with Redfield Associates, consultants, since 1983. She is chairman of the New York Rhodes Scholar Selection Committee, director of American Can, American Express, Chemical Bank, New York Stock Exchange, New York Telephone, chairman of the finance committee of the Council on Foreign Relations and member of the super secret American Council on Germany, which is said to be the behind the scenes government of West Germany; Robert E. Allen, who is director of AT&T, Pacific Northwest Bell, Manufacturers Hanover and the Manufacturers Hanover Trust; Henry H. Henley, Jr., chairman of Cluett Peabody, Clupak Corporation, General Electric, Home Life Insurance, Manufacturers Hanover Bank and the Manufacturers Hanover Trust, and trustee of Presbyterian Hospital, New York; James D. Robinson III, chairman of American Express, director of Shearson Lehman Hutton, Coca Cola, Union Pacific, Trust Company of Georgia, chairman of Rockefeller's Memorial Hospital for Cancer and Allied Diseases, Board manager of the Sloan Kettering Cancer Center, council member of Rockefeller University, chairman of the United Way, Council on Foreign Relations Business Council and the Business Roundtable; the epitome of the New York Establishment figurehead, Robinson was with Morgan Guaranty Trust from 1961 to 1968 as assistant to the president of the bank; Andrew C. Sigler, chairman of the key policy corporation, Champion Paper, director of Chemical New York, Cabot Corporation, General Electric and RCA.

Bristol-Myers is the 44th largest advertiser on the United States, with an annual expenditure of $344 million, mostly in television and advertising; this gives them a great deal of clout in dictating the content of programs. Bristol-Myers is now pushing its new tranquilizer, Buspar and its new anti-cholesterol drug, Questran, which it expects to gross at least $100 million a year each. The track record for anti-cholesterol drugs has revealed some disturbing side effects, such as liver damage and other "unforeseen" consequences.

Number 15 in world drug firm ranking is Beecham's Group of England, which specializes in human and veterinarian pharmaceuticals. Chairman of Beecham is Robert P. Bauman, who is also vice chairman of Textron, director of McKesson, another drug firm, and the media conglomerate, Capital Cities ABC. President of Beecham is Sir Graham Wilkins, director of Thorn EMI TV, Hill Samuel, the investment bankers, one of the Magic Seventeen merchant bankers licensed by the Bank of England, and Rowntree Mackintosh candy firm, as well as Courtauld's, the giant English textile firm which has close links with the British Secret Intelligence Service. Directors of Beecham are Lord Keith of Castleacre, who is chairman of Hill Samuel, investment bankers, director of Rolls Royce, British Airways, the *Times* Newspapers Ltd., and chairman of the Economic Planning Council, which has total power over businesses in England. Lord Keith was intelligence director of the Foreign Office before going into business. Another director of Beecham is Lord McFadzean of Kelvinside, who is chairman of Shell Transport and Trading, a Rothschild controlled firm, director of British Airways, Shell Petroleum and Rolls Royce. He is Commander of the Order of Orange Nassau, the super secret organization created to celebrate the establishment of William of Orange as King of England, and the subsequent chartering of the Bank of England. Beecham's American subsidiary does $500 million a year.

Number sixteen in world ranking is Bayer A. G. of Germany, one of the three spin-offs from I. G. Farben cartel after World War II. Set up under orders from the Allied Military Government, which was then dominated by General William Draper of Dillon Read investment bankers, Bayer is now larger than the original I. G. Farben. In 1977, Bayer bought Miles laboratories and Germaine Monteil Perfumes, in 1981, it bought Agfa Gevaert, another spinoff of American I. G. Farben, and in 1983 it bought Cutter Laboratories, a California firm which was famed as having been set up to protect the Rockefeller controlled drug firms in the great polio immunization wars. All of the faulty polio vaccine was said to have been produced by Cutter, freeing the Rockefeller firms from the threat of lawsuits. During the 1930s, Bayer operated Sterling Drug and Winthrop chemical companies in the United States as subsidiaries of the giant I. G. Farben cartel. Winthrop Chemical's president was George G. Klumpp, who had married into the J. P. Morgan family. Klumpp was chief of the drug division of the Food and Drug Administration in Washington from 1935-1941, when he became president of Winthrop Chemical. He had also been professor of medicine at Yale Medical School. A director of Winthrop, E. S. Rogers was physician at the Rockefeller Institute from 1932 to 1934, dean of the school of public health at the University of California at Berkley since 1946; Rogers had been consultant to the Secretary of War from 1941 to 1945. Laurance Rockefeller was also a director of Winthrop Chemical, showing the close connection between the Rockefellers and I. G. Farben. Rockefeller was also a director of McDonnell Aircraft, Eastern Air Lines, Chase Manhattan Bank, International Nickel, International Basic Economy Corporation, Memorial Hospital, and the Rockefeller Brothers Fund.

The number seventeen world ranked drug firm is Syntex, a firm prominent in agribusiness. Its founder-chairman, George Rosencrantz of Budapest, gives his present address as 1730 Parque Via Reforma, Mexico DF 10; he left the country after a bizarre kidnap scheme involving his wife. Chairman and president of Syntex is Albert Bowers, born in Manchester, England, a Fulbright fellow and member of the council at Rockefeller University; directors are Martin Carton, executive vice president of Allen and Company, Wall Street investment firm which was rumored for years to be the investment arm of Meyer Lansky's five hundred million dollar fortune from Mafia activities. Cartin is chairman of the finance committee of Fischbach Corporation, director of Rockcor Inc., Barco of California, Frank B. Hall & Company and Williams Electronics.

Other directors of Syntex include Dana Leavitt, chairman of Leavitt Management Corporation, director of Pritchard

Health Care, Chicago Title & Trust, United Artists, Transamerica, and chairman of Occidental Life Insurance; Leonard Marks, executive vice president of Castle & Cooke, the Hawaiian investment firm, director of the Times Mirror Corporation, Wells Fargo, Homestake Mining Company and California and Hawaii Sugar Company. Marks was Assistant Secretary of the Air Force from 1964-68. Also director of Syntex is a big name in banking, Anthony Solomon, now chairman of S. G. Warburg's Mercury International. Solomon was economist with the OPA when Richard Nixon began his career of government service there. Solomon then opened a canned soup firm in Mexico, Rosa Blanca, which he sold for many millions. He then returned to government service as an official of AID, president of the International Investment Corporation for Yugoslavia 1969-1972, was appointed Under Secretary for Monetary Affairs of the Treasury Department, 1977-1980, and succeeded Paul Volcker as president of the key money market bank, the Federal Reserve Bank of New York, when David Rockefeller moved Volcker up to become chairman of the Federal Reserve Board of Governors in 1980.

Solomon is also a director of Banca Commerciale Italiane.

Syntex is remembered for the mercurial rise in its stock when it began to dump vast amounts of condemned drugs in backward overseas countries. Its profits skyrocketed, as did its stock.

Number eighteen in world ranking is the former empire of Elmer Bobst, Warner-Lambert. It is the number nineteen advertiser in the United States, spending $469 million a year. Chairman of Warner-Lambert is Joseph D. Williams, who is also director of Warner-Lambert subsidiary, Parke-Davis, whose acquisition went through only because Bobst had secured the presidency for his friend Richard Nixon.

Williams is also a director of AT&T, J. C. Penney, Western Electric, Excello and Columbia University. He is chairman of the People to People Foundation. President of Warner-Lambert is Melvin R. Goodes, born in Canada, who was with the Ford Motor Company. Goodes was a fellow of the Ford Foundation and the Sears Roebuck Foundation.

Warner-Lambert, which was built into a drug empire by the many Bobst acquisitions, now features Listerine mouthwash (26.9% alcohol), Bromo Seltzer, Dentyne, Schick razors, Sloan's Linament, and Prazepan tranquilizer. Directors are B. Charles Ames, chairman of Acme Cleveland, the M. A. Hanna Corporation, Diamond Shamrock, and Harris Graphics; Donald L. Clark, chairman of Household International, the huge finance firm, Square D. Evanston Hospital and the Council on Foreign Relations; William R. Howell, chairman of J. C. Penney, director of Exxon and Nynex; Paul S. Morabito, director of Burroughs, Consumer Power, and Detroit Renaissance, the ill-fated experiment in "human rehabilitation" which poured billions into a Detroit rathole, and from which Henry Ford II resigned in disgust; Kenneth J. Whalen, director of American Motors, Combustion Engineering, Whirlpool and trustee of Union College; John F. Burdett, director of ACF Industries, General Public Utilities (which has sales of $2.87 billion a year). Chairman of ACF is the noted raider, Carl Icahn, who is chairman of the subsidiary IC Holding Company. Also directors of Warner-Lambert are Richard A. Cramer, Irving Kristol, kingpin of the neoconservative movement which centers around Jeane Kirkpatrick and the CIA; and Henry G. Parks, Jr., token black who founded Parks Sausage in Baltimore. He is now a director of W. R. Grace Company and Signal Company.

Other directors of Warner-Lambert are Paul S. Russell of the Harvard Medical School, Columbia College of Physicians and Surgeons, U.S. Navy, U.S. Public Health

Service, director of Sloan Kettering Cancer Center since 1974; and Edgar J. Sullivan, chairman of Borden, director of Bank of New York, director of F. W. Woolworth, professor and trustee of St. John's University. Sullivan is a Knight of Malta, director of the Council on Foreign Relations and the Atlantic Council. Sterling Drug, maker of Bayer's aspirin, and spinoff from the I. G. Farben cartel, is another important drug firm. Its chairman, W. Clark Wescoe, is a director of the Tinker Foundation, John Simon Guggenheim Foundation, Phillips Petroleum, and Hallmark Cards. He is chairman of the China Medical Board of New York, long the favorite charity of media tycoon Henry Luce. Wescoe is also trustee of the Samuel H. Kress Foundation and Columbia University, and controls billions in foundation funds. He is a director of the American Medical Association, the American College of Physicians, and the Council on Family Health. President of Sterling is John M. Pietruski, who was with Proctor and Gamble from 1954 to 1967, now director of Irving Bank, Associated Dry Goods (textile empire doing $2.6 billion a year); a later president, James G. Andress was with Abbott Laboratories; directors are Gordon T. Wallis, chairman of Irving Bank and Irving Trust, director of the Federal Reserve Bank of New York, Council on Foreign Relations, F. W. Woolworth, JWT Group, General Telephone and Electronics, Wing Hang Bank Ltd., and International Commercial Bank Ltd.; William E. C. Dear-den, who was chairman of Hershey Foods from 1964 to 1985, now with the Heritage Foundation, the pseudo-rightwing think tank run by the British Fabian Society; and Martha T. Muse, president of the very influential Tinker Foundation ($30 million). She is also director of Irving Bank, the American Council on Germany, ruling group of West Germany, Edmund A. Walsh School of Foreign Service, and Georgetown Center for Strategic and International Studies, all of which are the CIA preserves of veterans Evron and Jeane Kirkpatrick. She is also director of the Woodrow Wilson International Center and the Order of St. John of Jerusalem. Thus we find that Martha T. Muse is a veritable directory of top secret CIA worldwide operations.

The Tinker Foundation, like the Jacob Kaplan Fund, is one of the super secret organizations which funnels money to the CIA for covert activities too bizarre to be submitted to any government operations center. The secretary of the Tinker Foundation is Raymond L. Brittenham, who was born in Moscow, educated at the Kaiser Wilhelm Institute in Berlin. He was general counsel for ITT, whose German operations were headed by Baron Kurt von Schroder, personal banker to Adolf Hitler. Brittenham was senior vice president for law at ITT, Bell Tel, Belgian International, Standard Electric, vice president Standard Lorenz, Germany Harvard Law School, and partner of Lazard Freres investment bankers since 1980. Director of Tinker Foundation is David Abshire, White House confidant on sensitive intelligence matters. He is chairman of American Enterprise Institute, secret policy group headed by Jeane Kirkpatrick, and the Center for Strategic and International Studies. Abshire was U.S. Ambassador to NATO in Brussels, which serves as world headquarters and command center for the Rothschild World Order; Abshire headed the Reagan Transition team after Reagan's election to the White House; he also headed the National Security group, is on the administrative board of the Naval War College, the President's Foreign Intelligence Advisory Board and the influential International Institute of Strategic Studies.

Also director of Tinker Foundation is John N. Irwin II, educated at Oxford, partner of the Wall Street law firm, David Polk Wardwell until he moved on to Patterson Belknap. Irwin has been deputy assistant secretary of defense, internal security from 1957- 61, Under Secretary of State, Ambassador to France from 1970 to 1974. Irwin is a director of Morgan Guaranty Trust, IBM and the super secret 1925 F. Street Club in Washington. Vice chairman of the Tinker Foundation is Grayson Kirk, president of University of Wisconsin, president emeritus of University of Chicago, advisor to IBM, director of the Bullock Fund, the Asia Foundation, the French Institute, Lycee Francais, trustee of Money Shares, High Income Shares and the Hoover front, the Belgian-American Educational Foundation. Kirk is also recipient of the Order of the British Empire, St. John of Jerusalem, and is Commander of the Order of Orange- Nassau.

When Hoffman LaRoche made a strong bid for Sterling Drug in 1987, its cause was advanced by Lewis Preston, head of the J. P. Morgan empire, who was also banker for Sterling Drug. Publicity about his role caused his retirement for J. P. Morgan Company.

Sterling was then bought by Eastman Kodak through funding from the Rockefellers. Kodak banks at Chase Lincoln First Bank, which is wholly owned by Chase Manhattan Bank. Kodak does $10 billion a year; its chairman is C. Kay Whitmore, who is a director of Chase Manhattan Bank and Chase Manhattan National Corporation.

Directors of Kodak are Roger E. Anderson, former chairman of Continental Illinois Bank until it threatened to go under from mismanagement; he is now with Amsted Industries, a $700 million steel corporation. Anderson is also chairman of the Chicago branch of the Council on Foreign Relations. Other directors of Kodak are Charles T. Duncan, dean of the law school of Howard University, director of defense firm TRW, Proctor and Gamble and the NAACP Legal Defense Fund. A 32nd degree Mason, Duncan has long been active in black affairs, listing himself as assistant to now Supreme Court Justice Thurgood Marshall in the school desegregation case before the Supreme Court from 1953 to 1955. Juanita Kreps is also director of Kodak, she

251

was President Jimmy Carter's Secretary of Commerce; she is now director of RJR Industries and the New York Stock Exchange; she received the Stephen S. Wise award. Also on the board of Sterling are John G. Smale, chairman of Proctor and Gamble, director of General Motors; and Richard Mahoney, chairman of Monsanto Chemical Company.

Because they are active in similar chemical formulations, the leading chemical firms are also closely interlocked with the major drug producing firms. Richard Mahoney, director of Sterling Drug, is chairman of Monsanto Chemical, a $7 billion a year firm.

Mahoney claims he is seeking a twenty per cent return on equity for Monsanto this year. He is also director of Metropolitan Life Insurance Company, Centerre Bancorp, G. D. Searle. President of Monsanto is Earle H. Harbison, Jr., who was with the CIA from 1949 to 1967. Harbison is chairman of G. D. Searle, president of the Mental Health Association and director of Bethesda General Hospital and the St. Louis Hospital. Directors of Monsanto are Donald C. Carroll, dean of the Wharton School of Business; Richard I. Fricke, who was general counsel of the Ford Motor Company from 1957-1962, now chairman of the National Life Insurance Company and chairman of the Sentinel Group Funds; Howard A. Love, chairman of National Intergroup, formerly National Steel, director of Transworld Corporation and Hamilton Oil Corporation; Buck Mickel, construction tycoon, chairman of Daniel International Corporation which does over $1 billion a year, chairman RSI chairman of and Duke Power, president of the Fluor Corporation, vice chairman of J. P. Stevens, which is now undergoing a takeover bid, director of Seaboard Coast Line railroad.

Also director of Monsanto is William G. Ruckelshaus, who was deputy Attorney General of the United States and Assistant Attorney General in the Department of Justice Civil Department from 1969- 70, administrator of EPA from 1970 to 1973, served as Director of the FBI, senior vice president for law of the giant Weyerhauser Corporation, director of U.S. West and Pacific Gas Transmission; Stansfield Turner, who was director of the CIA from 1977 to 1981, a Rhodes Scholar, president of the Naval War College, Commander in Chief of NATO and the Second Fleet; C. Raymond Dahl, chairman of Crown Zellerbach, director of Bank America; John W. Hanley, former chairman of Monsanto, now director of Citibank, Citicorp and RJR Industries; Jean Mayer, son of the longtime chairman of Lazard Freres, Andre Mayer. Jean Mayer was born in Paris and is director of many organizations dealing with population studies; he was special consultant to the President of the United States from 1969-1970, and has been president of Tufts University since 1976, director of UNICEF and WHO; John S. Reed, chairman of Citibank, director of Philip Morris, United Technologies, Russell Sage Foundation, and the Sloan Kettering Cancer Center; John B. Slaughter, director of General Dynamics, Naval Electronic Lab at San Diego, NSF Missile Spec., and chancellor of the University of Maryland since 1982; he is active in a number of minority group organizations, Urban League, trustee Rensselaer Polytechnic Institute; Margaret Bush Wilson, a lawyer in St. Louis, treasurer of the NAACP and trustee of Washington University.

The close connection of the chemical industry and government intelligence is shown by the fact that Monsanto officers and directors include a CIA agent for twenty years, another former director of the CIA, former director of the EPA and the FBI and an engineer with General Dynamics, the nation's leading defense firm.

Although DDT was outlawed in this country, Monsanto continues to make handsome profits by shipping it overseas, particularly to countries in Latin America and Asia.

The eleven billion dollar a year Dow Chemical Corporation has directors including Carl Gerstacker, director of the Eaton Corporation. (Cyrus Eaton was a protege of John D. Rockefeller, long involved in pro-Soviet activities as organizer of the Pugwash Conference, which was directed by the KGB); Paul F. McCracken, economist for the Federal Reserve Bank of Minnesota from 1943- 48, professor of economics at the University of Michigan since 1948; McCracken was chairman of the Council of Economic Advisers from 1956-71, and has served on the President's Advisory Board of Economic Policy since 1981; Harold T. Shapiro, director of the Alfred P. Sloan Foundation, which funds the Rockefeller dominated Sloan Kettering Center, president of the University of Michigan, director of Ford Motor, Burroughs and Kellogg; Shapiro has served on the CIA panel since 1984. Although Dow was a family firm for many years, with Willard Dow as chairman, and three Dows on the board of directors, they are now all gone.

Mallinkrodt was another chemical firm long owned by one family; it is now a subsidiary of International Minerals and Chemical; there are no Mallinkrodts on its board. Directors are Jeremiah Milbank, a very influential New York family. He is president of the Milbank Fund, which is dominant in medical research; he is also treasurer of the Robert A. Taft School of Government, and vice president of the Boys Club of America, on which J. Edgar Hoover served for many years; Warren L. Batts, president of Dart Industries, director of the Mead Corporation, the First National Bank of Atlanta, Dart & Kraft and trustee of the American Enterprise Institute with Jeane Kirkpatrick; Frank W. Considine, chairman of National Can Corporation; Louis Fernandez, director of the Tribune Company in Chicago,

Encyclopedia Britannica, First Chicago National Bank, Allis Chalmers and Loyola University; Paul R. Judy, co-chairman Warburg Paribas Becker and director of Robert Bosch of North America; Rowland C. Frazee, chairman of the Royal Bank of Canada, director of Power Corporation of Canada, McGill University, and Portage Program for Drug Dependencies; James W. Glanville, was with Lazard Freres, now Lehman Brothers, director of the Halliburton Corporation; Thomas H. Roberts, Jr., chairman of DeKalb Agsearch, leading producers of hybrid corn, Continental Illinois bank, Board of Visitors Harvard University, president of St. Lukes Hospital, trust of Rush Medical College; Morton Moskin, lawyer with the Wall Street firm of White and Case, director of Crum & Forster.

For years, Mallinkrodt had a sweetheart deal with Memorial Hospital Sloan Kettering. One of the shadowy figures, now departed, who exercised a considerable influence behind the scenes was the man who set up this deal, M. Frederik Smith, a longtime Rockefeller associate who was director of Mallinkrodt. An indefatigable public relations man, Smith worked at Young & Rubicam, handled Bruce Burton's Congressional campaign, and masterminded the Wilkie bid for the presidency. Smith served as assistant to the President at the Bretton Wood conference and as assistant to the Secretary of the Treasury from 1924-44, representing the Rockefeller interests there. He also handled the public relations for Sloan Kettering Cancer Center, was a director of ABC and Simon and Schuster, handled public relations for the Book-of-the- Month Club and founded the United Nations Free World Association.

DuPont is another firm which for years was controlled by the DuPont family; they now have few representatives on its board.

Edgar Bronfman now has a 21% holding in its stock. A former director of DuPont was Donaldson Brown, who married Greta DuPont; he was director of the Federal Reserve Bank of New York, General Motors Acceptance Corporation and Gulf Oil. This $14 billion a year firm now has Andrew Brimmer, former Governor of the Federal Reserve Board, as director; he served as governor from 1966 to 1974.

A longtime rival of DuPont is Imperial Chemical Industries of England. It was founded by Alfred Mond, who became Lord Melchett. He formed agreements with I. G. Farben during the 1920s which allowed him to absorb British Dyestuffs and Nobel Industries in 1926. Its present chairman is Sir John Henry Harvey-Jones, director of Barclay's Bank. President of ICI is the 4th Baron Lord Melchett, Peter Mond, who finances the Greenpeace Environment Trust. Directors are Sir Robin Ibbs, a director of Lloyd's Bank, who serves as advisor to the Prime Minister. He is on the Council of the Royal Institute of International Affairs, the parent organization of our Council on Foreign Relations; Sir Alex A. Jarratt, who held many government offices from 1949 to 1970, including Minister of Power and Minister of State; he is now department chairman of the Midland Bank, and director of the Thyssen-Bornemitza Group; Sir Patrick Meaney, who is chairman of the Rank Organization, a moviemaking firm which was set up by the British Secret Intelligence Service; they imported a Hungarian, Rank, to run it for them and make anti-German movies in preparation for the start of the Second World War; Meaney is also a director of the Midland Bank. Also director of ICI is Sir Jeremy Morse, the chairman of Lloyd's; he was director of the Bank of England from 1965 to 1972, and is now president of the British Bankers Association; and also director of ICI is the media tycoon, Lord Kenneth Thomson, chairman of the Thomson Organization, which owns 93 newspapers in the United States; most Americans have never heard of him; he is also a director of IBM Canada and, Abitibi-Price, the newsprint giant. Donald C. Platten is also a director of Thomson Newspapers; he was formerly with the Federal Advisory Council of the Federal Reserve System; his daughter married Alfred Gwynne Vanderbilt.

Another chemical firm, Stauffer Chemical, is now a subsidiary of Cheseborough-Pond, a Rockefeller firm. Its chairman is Ralph E. Ward; he is a director of the Chase Manhattan Bank and the Chase Manhattan Corporation. The Rohm & Haas drug firm is in the Mellon Bank orbit, with prominent Philadelphia financiers as directors. They include G. Morris Dorrance, Jr., who is chairman of Corestates Financial Corporation, R. R. Donnelly Corporation, Federal Reserve Bank of Philadelphia, Provident Mutual Life Insurance, Banque Worms et cie of Paris and Verwaltungsrat John Berenberg, Gossler & Company. Dorrance is also a trustee of the University of Pennsylvania; Paul L. Miller, Jr., partner of Miller, Anderson & Sherrod; he is a director of Enterra Corporation, Hewlett Packard, Berwind Corporation, Mead Corporation and trustee of the Ford Foundation. Other directors are Robert E. Naylor, Jr., who was director of research for DuPont from 1956 to 1981; he is now with the Advanced Genetic Societies. Other drug companies include Schering-Plough, whose president, Richard J. Kogan, was with Ciba-Geigy; he is now director of the National Westminister Bank of the United States; directors are Virginia A. Dwyer, senior vice president for finance for AT&T; she is also a director of the Federal Reserve Bank of New York, Borden, and Eaton; Milton F. Rosenthal, was treasurer of Hugo Stinnes and now chairman of the leading gold dealer, Engelhard Corporation, and director of European American Banking Corporation. He is director of Salomon Brothers, Midatlantic Bank and Ferro Corporation; H. Guyford Spiver, chief scientist for the United States Air Force, president of Carnegie-Mellon

University, director of TRW ($5 billion a year defense contractor), science advisor to the President of the United States, holding many positions and offices in his *Who's Who* list; W. David Dance, director emeritus of General Electric, director of Acme Cleveland, A&P, Isek Corporation; Harold D. McGraw, Jr., chairman of the giant business publishing firm, McGraw Hill and director of Standard & Poor's, CPC International; I. W. van Gorkum, chairman of Trans Union Corporation, director of Champion International, IC Industries, Zenith Radio and Inland Steel; he is a member of the Bohemian Club.

Schering, a German firm, was seized by the Alien Property Custodian in 1942; it was sold by auction on March 6, 1952 by the Alien Property Custodian to a syndicate headed by Merrill Lynch, with Drexel & Company and Kidder Peabody joining in the deal.

Another drug firm, Burroughs Wellcome, is owned by the Wellcome Trust of England; its director is Lord Franks, a longtime trustee of the Rockefeller Foundation.

As was previously mentioned, Abbott Laboratories of Chicago, won recognition from the AMA for its products through adroit handling of the nation's preeminent quack, "Doc" Simmons. Its president Robert Schoellhorn, a director of Pillsbury and ITT; directors include K. Frank Austen, professor at the Harvard Medical School since 1960, chief physician at Beth Israel Hospital since 1980; he serves on many professional groups, including the Arthritis Foundation, and the American Board of Allergy and Immunology; Joseph V. Charyk, born in Canada, who was with Lockheed Aircraft, the space director and Under Secretary of the Air Force from 1959-1963; he was director of the communications satellite program; director of American Securities Corporation, Washington, D.C., Draper Laboratories, General Space Corporation, chairman of the

Communications Satellite Corporation and COMSAT Corporation. David A. Jones, chairman of the giant hospital firm, Humana Corporation, heads a firm with 17,000 employees which does $1.5 billion a year; he is also a director of Abbott Laboratories. The chairman of the executive committee of Abbott is Arthur E. Rasmussen, a director of Standard Oil of Indiana, trustee of the University of Chicago, which was established by a grant from John D. Rockefeller, trustee of the Field Foundation, and the International Rescue Committee, chairman of Household International and the Adler Planetarium; he is also a director of Amoco. Also director of Abbott Laboratories is Philip de Zulueta, a principal Rothschild operative in the British government for many years. De Zulueta is a close associate of Sir Mark Turner, who is chairman of the Rothschild firm Rio Tino Zinc. De Zulueta has been advisor to every Prime Minister of England since World War II; he was Private Parliamentary Secretary to Prime Minister Harold MacMillan. De Zulueta also has served for years as the private emissary between the Rothschilds of England and the Canada Bronfmans, who are their "cutouts" or front men in this hemisphere.

Another important world chemical firm is Unilever, founded in 1894; it is now headed by Lord Hunt of Tanworth, who held many important government positions from 1946 to 1973; he is also chairman of the Tablet Publishing Company, chairman of the top- secret Ditchley Foundation, (conduit for instructions between the governments of the United States and England), chairman of Banque Nationale de Paris and director of Prudential Corporation and IBM; vice chairman of Unilever is Kenneth Durham, who is chairman of Woolworth Holdings, Morgan Grenfell Holdings, United Technologies, Chase Manhattan Bank, Air Products and Chemicals, advisor to the New York Stock Exchange, director of British Aerospace and president of the Center for World Development and the Leverhulme

Trust. Unilever owns Lever Brothers in the United States; it bought Anderson Clayton Company in 1986, Thomas Lipton Company and Lawry's Foods.

The drug firms exercise a potent force in Washington through their lobbying activities. The chief lobbyist for the Pharmaceutical Manufacturers Association is Washington's highest-powered lobbyist, Lloyd Cutler. His mother was Dorothy Glaser; his sister Laurel married Stan Bernstein; she is now vice president of the public relations firm and advertising giant, McCann Erickson.

Cutler has been a partner of the Washington law firm Wilmer Cutler and Pickering since 1962. He was a counsel to the President from 1979 to 1981, and is a trustee of the prestigious Brookings Institution. A director of Kaiser Industries and American Cyanamid, Cutler was with the Lend Lease Administration, served as senior consultant to the Presidential Commission on Strategic Forces 1983, U.S. Group Permanent Court of Arbitration at the Hague 1984, and is a director of the Yale Development Board, the Foreign Policy Association and the Council on Foreign Relations. He is a member of the exclusive club, Buck's, in London and Lyford Cay, Nassau. He writes for the CFR magazine, *Foreign Affairs*. In an article, "To Form A Government," he complains that, "the structure of our constitution prevents us from doing significantly better." He urges that we should correct "this structural fault." The monopolists and their highly paid Washington lobbyists often find the Constitution a barrier to their plans; they cannot wait to get rid of it, because it is the only protection the citizens of the United States have left.

Hospital combines, as well as the drug firms, have become big business, and show close interlocking with major drug companies, Baxter Travenol, with $1.5 billion sales per year, interlocks with American Hospital Supply

Corporation, a $2.34 billion a year hospital operation. Both firms have the same chairman, Karl D. Bays; he is a director of Standard Oil of Indiana, the omnipresent Rockefeller connection. Bays is also a director of Northern Trust, Delta Airlines, IC Industries, Amoco, and trustee of Duke, Northwestern University and the Lake Forest Hospital. President of American Hospital Supply is Harold D. Bernthal, who is also director of Bucyars Erie Company, Butler Mfg., Bliss & Laughlin Industries and trustee of Northwestern University and Northwestern University Hospital. Directors of American Hospital Supply are Blaine J. Yarrington, executive vice president of Standard Oil of Indiana, director of the Continental Illinois Bank and trustee of the Field Museum of Natural History; Yarrington is also a director of Baxter Travenol. Other directors of American Hospital Supply are Harrington Drake, chairman of Colgate University, director of Corinthian Broadcasting System, Irving Bank, Irving Trust; Fred Turner, chairman of MacDonald's; Charles S. Munson, Jr., chairman of Air Reduction Corporation, Guaranty Trust, Cuban Distilling Company, National Carbide, Canada Dry, Reinsurance Corporation of New York, North British and Mercantile Insurance Company of London, trustee of the Taft School and Presbyterian Hospital; he was in the Chemical Warfare Service and served on the Army and Navy Munitions Board; also on the board of Baxter Travenol was William Wood Prince, a Chicago tycoon, president of F. H. Prince Company, director of Gaylord Freeman, director of Atlantic Richfield and trustee of the Aspen Institute of Humanistic Studies and trustee of Northwestern University.

Another giant hospital holding company, American Medical International of Beverly Hills, has seen its revenues climb from a mere $500 million a year to $2.66 billion in five years; it now has 40,000 employees. Chairman is Royce Diener; president is Walter Weisman; group vice president is Jerome Weisman. Directors include Henry Rosovsky, born in Danzig, Germany; he has been a director of the American Jewish Congress since 1975. Rosovsky was educated at Hebrew University, College of Jerusalem and Yeshiva University; he has been a professor at Harvard since 1965. Rosovsky is a member of the Harvard Corporation, director of Corning Glass and Paine Webber investment bankers.

Also director of AMI is Bernard Schriever, born in Bremen, Germany. As a general in the United States Air Force, Schriever was commander of the ICBM program from 1954 to 1959, Air Force Strategic Command from 1959-1966. He is now chairman of a contracting firm doing much government business in Washington, Schriever-McGee, since 1971. Schriever is also a director of Control Data, which operates under extensive Medicare and other government contracts, director of defense contractor Emerson Electric and transacts much of his business on the links of the exclusive Burning Tree Country Club, the historic haunt of defense contractors since President Eisenhower made it his favorite place of recreation.

Rocco Siciliano is also a director of AMI; he was with the National Labor Relations Board from 1953 to 1957, special assistant to President Eisenhower 1957-1959, Under Secretary of Commerce 1969-71, chairman of TICOR, 1971-1984, a leading California title insurance firm, which is now a subsidiary of Southern Pacific Siciliano was succeeded as chairman of this firm by Harold Geneen, former chairman of ITT. Siciliano is "of counsel" for the Washington lobbying firm, Jones, Day, Reavis and Pogue; he is also a director of the giant J. Paul Getty Trust and the Johns Hopkins University School of International Studies, which was founded by Owen Lattimore, (named by Senator Joe McCarthy as a leading Communist influence in the United States). Also director of AMI is S. Jerome Tamkin, a prominent Los Angeles stockbroker, head of Tamkin Securities and Tamkin Consulting Company.

The history of the pharmaceutical drug business has always been a chronicle of fraud, of preying on the fears of the uneducated and the gullible and taking advantage of the universal fears of the illness and death. The grand daddy of all nostrums is Goddard's drops, a bone distillate which was sold as a cure for gout in England in 1673. In 1711, Tuscarora rice was sold there as a cure for consumption. During some four thousand years of the practice of pharmaceutical prescriptions, many "cures" have been found to be worse than the disease. William Shakespeare warned, "In Physic there is Poison." Dr. R. R. Dracke, well known blood specialist in Atlanta, also issued a warning that "the following notable drugs may poison the marrow in the bones, decrease the production of white blood cells, may cause death and should be taken as medicine only with specific instruction from a well known doctor—amidopyrene, dinitrophenol (a diet drug), novaldine, antipyrene, sulphanilamide, sedormid and salvarsen."

Physicians have warned that no acetanilid is safe, because all coal tar derivatives are powerful heart depressants. Rorer Pharmaceuticals makes Ascriptin, and television advertisements have been urging men to take an aspirin or aspirin product daily "to protect their heart." The attorneys general of Texas and New York have requested drug firms to halt the claim that aspirin may prevent heart attacks in men; it also reduces fever and makes it difficult for a physician to correctly diagnose pneumonia.

The William S. Merrell Company, merged with Vick Chemical, marketed thalidomide as the "tranquilizer of the future." It guaranteed control of unpleasant symptoms during pregnancy.

Unfortunately, the children of mothers who took it were born without arms or legs; some had flippers for arms. 60 Minutes recently presented a twenty-five year update on

English victims of thalidomide, carefully avoiding any treatment of American victims. The program showed the astounding courage of the victims, who tried to carry on daily life, while the reporters seemed hard put to keep from bursting into laughter at the strange beings who rolled around like human eggs, maneuvering frantically to stay right side up. CBS also avoided any mention of the names of the manufacturers or distributors of thalidomide, although a typical operation of their brand of "adversary journalism" would have been to thrust a microphone into the face of the firm's chairman, and demand to know why they didn't realize this was a dangerous drug. CBS depends heavily on advertising revenues from the pharmaceutical manufacturers, and they are not about to offend their best customers.

William S. Merrell also produced MER/29, which was advertised as breakthrough in anticholesterol drugs. It was soon found that MER/29 caused dermatitis, changing color of hair, loss of sex drive and a condition known as "alligator skin." In 1949, Parke- Davis' chloromycetin was hailed as the new wonder drug. Several doctors were persuaded to give it to their children, who then died of leukemia. 75% of the cases of aplastic anemia resulting from the administration of chloromycetin were fatal. Dr. H. A. Hooks of El Paso lost his seven and a half year old son, after he had been assured by a Parke-Davis representative that the drug was safe. In December 1963, a Washington grand jury indicted Richard Merrell and chairman William S. Merrell for falsifying date to the FDA on MER/29. They filed a "no contest" plea and on June 4, 1964 were fined the maximum fine, $80,000. Parke-Davis defense counsel was a former federal judge from 1957 to 1960, Lawrence Walsh, who is now much in the news as the White Knight who is prosecuting political figures on vague charges of malfeasance.

After an oral contraceptive pill was found to cause severe reactions, the American Medical Association put great pressure on Dr. Roger Hegeberg, Assistant Secretary of HEW and the Secretary of HEW, Finch, claiming they were "over-emphasizing dangers"; the warning on the pill was then cut from 600 words to only 96 much milder words; this warning was increased by Secretary Finch himself of April 7, 1970 to 120 words of warning, which was released personally by Finch. The pill was then found to cause fatal blood clotting, heart attack and cancer. The behaviour of the AMA in this instance contrasted strangely with its violent attacks for many years on "quacks," who it protested were the real dangers to the public.

Hoffman LaRoche marketed an intravenous drug, Versed, which was linked to forty deaths in two years by FDA studies. Richter's definitive work, "Pills, Pesticides and Profits," notes that a U.S. company, Velsicol, sold three million pounds of a pesticide, Phosvel (leptophos), which had never been approved by the EPA. Velsicol exported it to thirty countries. It causes extensive damage to the nervous system. In Egypt, it killed one hundred water buffalo and poisoned dozens of farmers. Velsicol is a subsidiary of Northwest Industries, a three billion dollars a year operation in Chicago whose chairman is longtime rail magnate, Ben Heinemann, a trustee of the University of Chicago, and the First Chicago Corporation. Directors of Northwest Industries are James E. Dovitt, director of Hart, Schaffner and Marx, president of Mutual of New York, and director of MONY; he is also a director of National Can. Other directors of Northwest are William B. Graham, chairman of Baxter Travenol Drug Company, also a trustee of the University of Chicago, director of Deere, Field Enterprises, Bell & Howell and Borg-Warner; National Council of U.S. China Trade; Thomas S. Hyland, vice president of Standard & Poor's; Gaylord Freeman, director of Baxter Travenol and Atlantic Richfield; James F. Bere, chairman of Borg-Warner, director of Abbott Laboratories, Time, Inc., Hughes Tool Company and Continental Illinois Bank.

After TRIS, a fire-retardant chemical used in clothing, was banned in the United States, after years of enthusiastic advertising that it would save thousands of children from death by fire each year, the U.S. Consumer Product Safety Commission banned it in 1977. 2.4 million TRIS treated garments were then exported to the Third World. In 1977, the FDA removed dipyrene from the market. It had been found to cause severe blood disorders, interfering with the white blood cell function; it was then sold widely in Latin America with no warning.

Cloquinol, a drug used to treat amoebic dysentery, produced by Ciba-Geigy in 1934 (Batero Vioform and Mexon) was found to cause a nerve disorder. Seven hundred Japanese died from taking it, after 11,000 cases of SMON, subacute myelic optic neuropathy. Ciba-Geigy then paid a settlement to some 1500 victims and survivors. Hoechst marketed an analgesic said to be like aspirin, aminopyrein and dipyrene. It was found to cause anemia and was banned in the United States, but continued to be sold in Latin America and Asia. Chlorophenicol (chloromycetin) also is still sold in Latin America and Asia. Travellers are warned to beware of drugs in foreign countries which have long been banned in the United States.

The artificial sweetener, aspartame (Nutrasweet) has now flooded the American market. It earned $750 million for its producers in 1987, although it has come under attack as a cause of brain seizures. The debate about aspartame has been going on for thirteen years; more Congressional hearings have now been scheduled. Meanwhile, Burroughs Wellcome hopes to make millions with its new drug for AIDS, AZT. It is said to prolong the life of AIDS victims from six months to two years. This firm is owned by the Wellcome Trust, of which Lord Franks, a director of the Rockefeller Foundation, is director.

Tranquilizers continue to be big business. Roche Labs (Hoffman LaRoche) continues to push its No. 1 seller, Valium, while promoting its other sellers, Librium, Limbitrol, Marplan, Noludar, Tractan, Clonpin and Dalmane. Roche also produces Matulane, which is used in cancer therapy. This drug causes leukopenia, anemia, and thrompenia, with side effects of nausea, vomiting, stomatitis, dysphagia, diarrhea, pain, chills, fever, sweating, drowsiness, tachycardia, bleeding and leukemia. If an alternative health care practitioner ever dared to offer such a drug to the public, he would be incarcerated for life. We all know how dangerous "quacks" are to your health. Roche's medical director, Dr. Bruce Medd, hails these drugs as boons to mankind. Listen to his rhapsodizing, "Unlike quack remedies, which are neither tested nor scientifically proven, Roche products stand for quality and efficiency. We at Roche join the fight against medical quackery and health fraud." Despite Dr. Medd's assurances, the Office of Technology Assessment of the U.S. Government states that 95% of the drugs on the market have not been proven to work. Indeed, this writer has never heard of any "quack" remedy producing even a fraction of the harmful side effects as those listed above as caused by Matulane, Dr. Medd's pride and joy.

Another firm offering "proven" drugs is Smith, Kline Beck- man, which made its initial millions from peddling the drug known as "speed" through prescriptions from doctors, the notorious Dexedrine and Dexamil. Executives of Smith, Kline Beckman have pled guilty to 34 charges of covering up 36 deaths and cases of severe kidney damage in patients using their drug Selocrin, which was finally removed from the market. Dr. Sidney M. Wolfe, in his Health Letter, July,

1986 noted that Eli Lilly of Indiana and Smith Kline Corporation of Philadelphia pled guilty to criminal charges of failing to notify promptly the FDA of deaths and serious injuries to people using their drugs. Lilly's Oraflex, an arthritis drug, was on the market three months and used by 600,000 Americans before it was withdrawn due to its side effects. Smith Kline's high blood pressure, Selacryn, sold 300,000 prescriptions in eight months.

Pfizer withheld information from the FDA about Feldene (pyroxicam, an arthritis drug), despite deaths and harmful side effects in other countries. McNeil's Suprol, approved in 1985 as an oral analgesic was found to cause kidney damage. Orudis (jetoprofen), Wyeth's arthritis drug, increased the incidence of ulcers. Merital (nomigensine), an antidepressant produced by Hoechst, was approved by the FDA in December 1984, but had to be taken off the market in January 1986, because of fatal reactions, including hemolytic anemia. Wellbutrin (buproprion) was found to cause convulsions in women and was removed from the market in March 1986.

An officially approved "standard of care" drug for treatment of cancer of the colon is based on the use of a highly toxic chemical, 5- F-U, despite reports in prestigious medical journals that it doesn't work. It continues to be widely used, perhaps because the American Cancer Society owns 50% of 5-F-U. Ciba-Geigy of Switzerland has found an increasing market in the U.S. public school system for its drug Ritalin, which through some alchemy has now become the principal means of controlling "hyperactive" (read healthy) school children. Social workers had coined a new term ADD (attention defect disorder), which could be "controlled" by 20 mg tablets of Ritalin in sustained release capsules. Aided by the education establishment, which has a propensity for any drug or chemical addition to the educational process, Ritalin has had a 97% increase in use since 1985. Students are forced to take the drug, or to face immediate expulsion from school. The *Wall Street Journal,* January 15, 1988, noted that a number of suits have been filed against schools by anxious parents concerning the forced use of Ritalin. The Georgia Board of Medical Examiners is now looking into the skyrocketing use of Ritalin in the schools in Atlanta's affluent suburbs. A student now on trial for murder has entered the defense that he was on Ritalin.

Pesticides persist in being even more dangerous than insects.

Lindane, (Gammelin 20), produced by Hooker Chemical, a Rockefeller connected firm, causes dizziness, brain disease, convulsions, muscle spasms, and leukemia. For years, the FDA waged a battle against Shell Oil's pesticide strips, which contain lindane. These strips and other vaporizers continuously emit lindane, and are widely used in restaurants, even though it had been established that lindane not only contaminates any food substance, but also any container for food which is not metal. Although these tests were concluded in 1953, the Pesticides Regulator continued to allow their use for another sixteen years! FDA reports showed that Shell Chemical Company's No Pest Strips continually release Vapone 3, the lindane formulation. The Agriculture Department strictly forbade their use in meat processing plants, but the enterprising manufacturer then peddled them to restaurants. From 1965 to 1970, the U.S. Public Health Service released warnings that Shell No Pest Strips were dangerous to use in sleeping rooms of the elderly or of small children. Dr. Roy T. Hansberry, executive of Shell Chemical, which subsidized Shell Development, served on the special Agricultural Department seven member task force to study pesticide registration procedures. Shell had registered 250 pesticide products. Hansberry's personal clearance to serve on this task force carried the unsigned note, "The Agricultural Registration Service does not have, or know of, any official business with the persons, firms or institutions with which Dr. Hansberry has other financial interests. which might conflict or constitute a conflict of interest."

Dr. Mitchell A. Zaron, assistant health commissioner, also served as a consultant to Shell Chemical, and owned Shell Oil stock. He issued reports which purportedly showed Vapona as so safe that it required no warnings for infants, or for old or sick persons. At a meeting of the Public Health Service, he endorsed the use of Vapona strips. John S. Leary, Jr., research division chief staff officer for Pharmacology, overruled the department's objection to the original Shell registration of Vapona, in 1963, and continued to support the use of Vapona, until in 1966, when he resigned to join Shell Oil Company. It is estimated there have been thousands of victims each year suffering from exposure to Shell No Pest Strips.

Another pesticide, parathion, which was manufactured by Monsanto and Bayer A. G., also has had baneful side effects. The pesticide, malathion, used in Pakistan in 1976, poisoned 2,500 persons, many of whom died. And DDT, as we have noted, long after its ban in the United States, continues to find a ready market overseas, much to the profit of Mansanto, its producer.

In 1975, investigators found that two widely prescribed drugs, Adactone and Flagyl, produced by G. D. Searle Company, caused cancer in test animals. They had annual sales of $17.3 million. The firm had given FDA fraudulent data and destroyed records of tumors in mice caused by these drugs.

A Consumers Protective Message, issued from Washington March 15, 1962, noted that since 1938, manufacturers had to demonstrate the efficacy of a medicine to the government before marketing it. However, the regulation contained a significant loophole—there was no stated requirement for a demonstration of its efficacy, or to furnish evidence that the drug "will live up to its claim of its labelling." The Message stated, "There is no way of measuring the needless suffering, the money innocently squandered and the protraction of illnesses resulting from the use of such inefficient drugs." In 1962, Congress enacted the Kefauver-Harris amendments requiring evidence of efficacy. The evidence was to be judged by the Food and Drug Administration Bureau of Medicine, but the post of chief of that bureau was vacant because Bois-feuillet Jones, special assistant for medical affairs at HEW, blocked the appointment of Dr. Charles D. May, a distinguished physician who had testified at the Kefauver hearings on the methods of the pharmaceutical manufacturers in promoting prescription drugs. Dr. May had testified that the payola and other promotions amounted to three and a half times as much as the cost of all the educational programs in our medical schools. Jones "won the confidence of the pharmaceutical industry by blocking the appointment of Dr. May" according to a report in *Drug Research Reports,* June, 1964. Instead of Dr. May, Jones chose Dr. Joseph F. Sadusk, Jr. who did everything he could to thwart the efficacy legislation, according to testimony before the Senate Committee on Government Operations. Sadusk later became a vice-president of Parke-Davis. Sadusk had prevented the recall of Parke-Davis' antibiotic drug Chloramphenicaol, which had resulted in blood toxicity and leukopenia, before he was offered the vice-presidency of Parke- Davis. He was succeeded as medical director of the FDA by Dr. Joseph M. Pisani at the Bureau of Medicine. Pisani left to work for the Proprietary Association of Drug Manufacturers. The next head of the Bureau of Medicine later became a top executive at Hoffman LaRoche. Dr. Howard Cohn, former head of the FDA medical evaluation board, was offered a job at Ciba-Geigy which he accepted. Dr. Harold Anderson, chief of the FDA drug division, was given a job with Winthrop Drug Company. Morris Yakowitz found that his experience at FDA made him eligible for a job at Smith Kline and French drug firm. Allan E. Rayfield, who had been director of Regulatory Compliance, accepted a position with Richardson-Merrell, Inc.

Thus we find that the revolving door has long been a characteristic of government regulation of the pharmaceutical industry. Surgeon General Leonard Scheele became president of Warner-Lambert Research Labs; FDA Commissioner Charles C. Edwards is now listed as senior vice-president of Becton Dickinson, a large medical supply firm. Although it is hardly a household word, it does one billion dollars a year in the medical field. Its chairman, Wesley Howe, is founding chairman of the Health Industry Manufacturers Association. FDA Commissioner James L. Goddard became chairman of the board at Ormont Drug and Chemical Company, whose president is George Goldenberg. The previously mentioned Joseph Sadusk, the top physician at FDA, after accepting a position as vice-president of Parke-Davis, later was named its president.

One might think that these gentlemen had left FDA only to find more pleasant working conditions, which were notably depressing at FDA. Dr. Richard Crout, test director at the FDA Bureau of Drugs, addressed the Pharmaceutical Manufacturers Association in 1976 as follows: "There was open drunkenness by several employees which went on for months. crippled by what some peopled called the worst personnel in government. There was intimidation internally by people, people tittering in corners, throwing spitballs; I am describing physicians, people who would slouch down in a chair, not respond to questions, moan and groan with sweeping gestures." (from New England *Journal of Medicine*, May 27, 1976).

One may ask why a government department composed of professionally educated scientists and physicians would tolerate such working conditions. The answer is that that Medical Monopoly wanted these conditions and saw to it that they prevailed at the FDA, so as to drive away sincere, dedicated government servants who wanted only to do their job, who desired to protect the public from dangerous drugs. It seems that the most dangerous drugs are also the most profitable, because they produce dramatic, easily seen results. Unfortunately, they also tend to produce such dramatic side effects as kidney and brain damage, or sudden death.

The drug manufacturers are adept at organizing influential lobbying groups in Washington, of which the public remains unaware. Some ninety-six companies, including Dow, Monsanto, Hoffman LaRoche and many others, put up five thousand dollars each per year to support the Council of Agricultural Science and Technology and the Institute of Food Technology, groups which systematically mislead the public about the dangers of cancer- causing food additives. They are able to minimize and weaken the frequent attempts by Congressmen to expose the dangers of many of these additives. It is all part of the game of public relations.

In the 1950s, Senator Estes Kefauver was one of the nation's most influential politicians. It seemed certain that he was headed for the White House. However, due to a flood of complaints from his constituents about the drug industry practices of gouging the elderly and producing dangerous drugs, Kefauver scheduled comprehensive hearings before the Senate on the widespread abuses committed by the Medical Monopoly. He even called his Subcommittee, the Senate Anti-Monopoly Subcommittee. These hearings, held during 1959 and 1960, revealed that Schering had markups of 1,118% on its drug, predisone and that other drug manufacturers routinely showed profits of from 10,000% to 20,000% on their drugs. The outcome of these hearings was the government recommendations for the promotion of "generic," or cheaper non-brand-name, drugs for mass sales of the same drugs at cheaper prices. Ostensibly a move to curb the excessive profits of the drug companies, the net result was that these companies showed vast increases in their volume of sales, with corresponding increase in profits. A more tragic result was that these hearings proved to be Senator Kefauver's political Waterloo. Stung by the publicity and the criticism which resulted from the hearings, the word went out from the Medical Monopoly, which we have shown, is not merely the officers and employees visible to the public, but the shadowy figures in the background, (many of them aliens, who control millions of shares in these companies through the practice of "street names," concealing their power), that "Kefauver is through." When he inaugurated his campaign for the presidency, he found that funds had mysteriously dried up. Without money, his candidacy was doomed. Disconsolate, he abandoned his campaign for the White House and later died, some said of a broken heart. Political figures got the message; there have been no repeats of the Kefauver hearings on the abuses of the drug industry. Individual products, such as the current furore over aspartame, may come under Congressional scrutiny, but the overall operations of the Drug Trust remain immune from Congressional investigation.

Meanwhile, the drug companies roar ahead with vast sales and record profits on their new drugs. Squibb's Capoten, a hypertension drug, could reach $900 million in sales this year, almost a billion dollars from a single product! Merck expects Vesoten, another hypertension drug, to reach $720 million in sales this year. In 1987, Merck had thirteen products in eight therapeutic classes which reached sales of more than $100 million each. Because of this high volume, the cost of production had dropped steadily for the major drug firms, an average of a 15% drop since 1980. In effect, this has meant an increase in profits of 15% from this single factor.

In 1987, Syntex reported that 53% of its sales volume of $1.1 billion came from just two products, Noprosyn and Ahaprox.

Business Week, January 11, 1988, predicts "another gold mine for U.S. Drugmakers." However, this gold mine would be nothing more than another dry shaft were it not for the continuing increasing prescription for these drugs to their patients by U.S. physicians. The Medical Monopoly's weak link is that it is almost totally dependent on doctors and hospital personnel to promote its profitable items. The $18 to $20 million expenditure required to get a new drug through the testing period of from three to twelve years is not intended to protect the public from "dangerous" new drugs. It is needed to protect the Drug Trust as long as possible, affording them the necessary time to milk their present drugs for as much sales as possible before they are replaced by newer competing drugs. It is called "protecting market share" in the business world. It would be called a violation of the anti-trust laws were the drug firms not immune from prosecution under these statutes.

As the stock market slowly recovered from the well planned and executed Black Monday, the stock market crash of October 19, 1987, the drug firms are more than holding their own, rewarding the astute monopolists who bought in at the bottom of the market.

Typical of investment policies of insurance companies are those of Equitable Life, which in 1987, had 7.8% of its assets invested in the stock of drug manufacturers, including $13 million in Marion Labs, $4 million in Merck, $7 million in Syntex and $4 million in Upjohn. Another 5.8% of its investments were in the stock of the very profitable hospital supply firms.

No chronicle of the world's important drug firms would be complete without relating the connection between drug firms and the world drug operation known as "Dope, Inc." It began with a small group of international financiers, headquartered in London, who officiated in the setting up of an "American" intelligence service, which was initially known as the Office of Strategic Services during World War II. This organization was set up under the close supervision of the British Secret Intelligence Service and was later disbanded by President Truman, who was highly suspicious of its operations. The OSS then went underground at the State Department as a "research group" working on "behavioural theory." It was led by one Evron Kirkpatrick, whose wife, Jeane Kirkpatrick, is a director of the Rockefeller financed Trotskyite group, League for Industrial Democracy and who is frequently touted as "a great anti-Communist," the catch being that all good Trotskyites are vehemently opposed to the Moscow branch of the Communist Party. They still mourn the passing of their leader, Leon Trotsky, who was murdered by a Stalinist agent in Mexico City in 1940. The Kirkpatrick group then resurfaced as "the Central Intelligence Agency," headed by Allen Dulles, a partner in the Schroder Bank, the bank which had handled Adolf Hitler's personal bank account. Dulles' brother, John Foster Dulles, was then Secretary of State under President Eisenhower.

Whatever interest the CIA may have had in "intelligence," it soon became clear that its primary interest was in the realization of the enormous profits to be made in the international dope trade.

Because British fortunes in the early nineteenth century had been founded in this trade, it was logical that the SIS operatives who set up our OSS, later CIA, would have been programmed to go into this business. It later became known by the inside sobriquet, "the Company," meaning, of course, an enterprise in which one became engaged for profit. The excuse advanced to justify going into this business was that a "stingy" Congress refused to advance enough money to the CIA to finance its covert operations; therefore a loyal CIA agent would do whatever possible to aid "the Company" to raise funds needed for this work. In fact, some of its most active agents, such as Edwin Wilson, suddenly wound up owning six million dollar estates in the developing area off the Washington Beltway, a certain indication that there was indeed a lot of money coming in from somewhere. What is the present magnitude of the CIA world drug operation? Lt. Col. Bo Gritz, who has thirty years of distinguished service with the United States Army Special Forces, testified before the House Foreign Affairs Committee International Narcotic Task Force that 900 tons of heroin and opium would enter the free world in 1987, the source being Southeast Asia and the Golden Triangle. Col. Gritz had been to Asia a number of times to confer with one of Asia's largest drug producers, Khun Sa. Khun Sa then laid the blame for the world drug operation squarely at the door of some well known CIA operatives, including Theodore Shackley, who served as chief of station for the CIA in Laos from 1965 to 1975. Khun Sa stated that Shackley had worked closely with Mao Se Hung, who was then the leading drug smuggler in Southeast Asia. Another colleague of Shackley was a "civilian" named Santos Trafficante. Trafficante had long been a leading figure in the Mafia, and had been called before Congress to testify about a possible attempt on the life of Castro in Cuba. When the Communist regime took over, the Mafia lost an empire of gambling and prostitution in Havana and other cities. They sought revenge. Trafficante was commissioned by Meyer Lansky, the Moneybags of the Syndicate, to get rid of Castro. Whether the attempt failed, or as is more likely, the Mafia came to an understanding with Castro about the dope traffic, is not yet known. Trafficante then became heavily involved in the Pacific area of the drug traffic, becoming a go-between for the Nugan Hand operation, the drug bank in Australia and the Golden Triangle.

Another prominent personality identified by Khun Sa and others as active in the drug trade was Richard Armitage, whose drug operations began during the Vietnam War. He later moved to the U.S. Embassy in Bangkok. From 1975 to 1979, according to witnesses, he used his embassy position to carry on drug operations. He then left that post, establishing the Far East Trading Corporation in Bangkok. Armitage was later appointed by President Reagan as Assistant Secretary of Defense in charge of International Security Affairs, reporting directly to the Secretary of Defense, Casper Weinberger. Business tycoon Ross Perot then learned of Armitage's history. He went to the White House, demanding that Armitage be fired. He talked to George Bush, former head of the CIA, who gave him the brushoff by sending him to FBI Director William Webster (shortly afterwards, Webster was quietly appointed head of the CIA). Webster refused to act on Perot's complaints, which opened the door for his appointment to the CIA post. Meanwhile, Weinberger, fearful that the role of the Defense Department in the drug scandal was about to unfold, hastily resigned. He was succeeded by Frank Carlucci, who was then serving as National Security Advisor, and who was well versed in the entire operation. Carlucci personally ordered Perot to drop his crusade against Armitage. Because Perot's fortune had been built on huge government contracts, he had no choice but to back off. Other personages involved were General Richard Secord, who surfaced as a figure in the Iran-Contra affair, who had boasted of flying plane loads of gold to Southeast Asia to pay off the drug smugglers.

The daytime soap opera known as the Iran-Contra affair was made to order for the secretive operatives of the CIA. They delighted in leading the obtuse members of Congress on one wild goose chase after another, while the real story remained untold. It was chef's surprise, a culinary delight of drugs, the sale of arms to belligerents, and money, well seasoned with political sauce, stirred with various commitments to the State of Israel by leading Washington politicians, and topped with luscious Swiss bank accounts. In fact, the Iran Contra affair was the logical culmination of the longtime involvement of the Rockefeller interests and the Drug Trust in pro-Communist activity. John D. Rockefeller himself had tucked the sum of $10,000 in cash into Leon Trotsky's pocket before seeing him off to start the Bolshevik Revolution in Russia. The Trotskyite Socialist Workers Party which was left behind to subvert the United States, was operating under the name of the Socialist Workers Party. It was then given the cover name of League for Industrial Democracy. Thus the Drug Trust, while maintaining the Stalinist Communist government in Russia, simultaneously maintained a Communist backup regime in the United States, the Trotskyite movement, in case the Stalinist regime should fall.

Noticeably irked by this competition, Stalin sent an agent Mexico to eliminate his rival, whom he had previously exiled, realizing that Trotsky was still too popular in Russia to be murdered there.

The Trotsky organization now had its political martyr. During the 1950s, it quietly placed its members in power in the media, the universities and the government, replacing, in most instances, the incumbent Stalinist hardliners. The Stalinists in Washington who had surrounded Roosevelt and Truman were gradually replaced with "neoconservatives," that is, hard-line anti-Moscow ideologues, who later added to their masquerade by additional and impressive noms de plume, such as "the Hard Right," "the New Right," "the Religious Right," or, in some instances, merely as "conservatives." None other than the Hollywood man on the white horse, Ronald Reagan, rode into power in 1980 on a tide of "neoconservatism." His principal backing came from the CIA, which by then was only a mouthpiece for the neoconservatives, and its house organ, the *National Review,* whose editor, William Buckley, boasted that the only job he had ever had was with the CIA. Jeane Kirkpatrick, of the Rockefeller financed League for Industrial Democracy, became the spokesman for the new policy, while Reagan's entire team was dominated by the Hoover Institution, whose two senior fellows, Sydney Hook and Seymour Martin Lipset, were on the board of LID. Thus David Rockefeller maintained close liason with the Stalinist Communists in Moscow, while other Rockefeller interests directed the "anti-Communist" stance of the Reagan regime. It was a classic Hegelian operation of thesis and antithesis, with the still unresolved synthesis yet to come. The power of the LID lay in its domination of the CIA and its total commitment to the State of Israel as the world headquarters of the Trotskyite Communist movement. Thus Elliott Abrams, son-in-law of the Israeli propagandist Norman Podhoretz, who was editor of the American Jewish Committee organ, *Commentary,* was appointed by Reagan to direct the Contra operation in Nicaragua, a classic standoff between the Stalinist regime in Managua and Trotskyite directed rebels in the hills.

The drug involvement in this operation should surprise no one, because the Rockefeller interests, having established the American Drug Trust, had long been active not only in ethical drugs but in unethical ones as well. The contra affair not only threatened to blow the lid off the Iran Connection; it endangered the Israeli Connection, the Swiss Connection, and the Rockefeller Connection as well. The danger was averted by astute maneuvering of the docile congressmen, and by adroit manipulation of the media to focus on Col. Oliver North and Admiral Poindexter, to the exclusion of their controllers. Thus a "crusade against Communism," a noble effort to contain the Communists a la George Kennan, to be financed with "dirty" money from the sale of drugs, was at last revealed to be the same old crew of CIA agents peddling their drugs and laundering their money in various parts of the world. (The present writer is now researching a book which will document all of these operations.)

The CIA drug connection was not only deeply rooted in the quest for easy profits, but also in the concurrent plan to achieve total control over the people of the world by the masters of the Drug Trust. Thus Bowart states, "The Cryptocracy is a brotherhood reminiscent of the ancient secret societies, with rites of initiation and indoctrination programs to develop in its loyal membership the special understanding of its mysteries. It has secret codes and oaths of silence which reinforce the sense of elitism necessary for the maintenance of its strict loyalty." The present writer has described some of these secret rites in "The Curse of Canaan."

The emphasis on drugs and experimentation which originated with the German allopathic school of medicine, and which was brought to this hemisphere by Illuminati initiates such as Daniel Coit Gilman, was the first step in transforming the entire medical practice of the United States from a patient-oriented, healing process to a totally different approach, in which the patient became an instrument to be manipulated for the benefit of various other programs, mainly experimental science. This had been typified by Dr. J. Marion Sims, the "mad doctor" responsible for setting up what is now the Rockefeller controlled Memorial Hospital Sloan Kettering Cancer Center in New York. This total commitment to "Science" also guided and inspired the CIA drug programs, Projects Bluebird, Artichoke, MK Ultra, and MK Delta, in which some 139 drugs were used on unsuspecting victims, the substances abused including cannabis, LSD, Scopolamine, Sodium Amytal, Chloral Hydrate (the knockout drops of the Old West), ergot, cocaine, morphine and heroin.

The CIA drug story begins in 1943, when the organization was still known as the OSS. A Dr. Albert Hoffmann was experimenting in the Sandoz Laboratories in Switzerland (Sandoz was then controlled by the Warburg family). Although Sandoz has been manufacturing a substance known as LSD, or lysergic acid, since 1938, it had only been used in experiments with monkeys. A later form of this substance, LSD-25, produced amazing psychotropic effects, as Dr. Hoffmann accidentally discovered, when he absorbed a small quantity of rye fungus, the base for the drug, while he was working. This happened during August of 1943, at the height of the Second World War. Dr. Hoffmann later reported, "There surged upon me an uninterrupted stream of fantastic images of extraordinary plasticity and vividness and accompanied by an intense kaeleidoscopic-like play of colors ... I thought I was dying or going crazy." This was the first "trip," the precursor of millions of such experiences by drug cultists. By 1958, Dr. Hoffmann had expanded his interests to Mexican mushrooms and mescaline, both of which then became very popular among leading bankers in New York, and among prominent Hollywood personalities.

At the time of the discovery of LSD, Allen Dulles was posted in Switzerland, as though by precognition. It was under his leadership that the CIA became transformed into the foremost operation of Dope, Inc. He was then engaged in various activities with officials of the Nazi regime. To this day, no one has been able to ascertain whether he was trying to preserve the Hitler regime, or to overthrow it. The most likely assumption is that he was trying to preserve it to a point, lest the war end too soon for the profit-minded munitions makers, but at the same time to prevent any sort of victorious ending for his Nazi cohorts. The notes of Gotterdammerung had already been sounded. Dulles' association with the Hitler regime went back to a fateful meeting in Cologne in 1933, when he and his brother, John Foster Dulles, assured Hitler the money would be forthcoming to guarantee the fruition of his goals as he had set them forth in "Mein Kampf." Allen Dulles later became a director of the Schroder Bank, which handled Hitler's personal bank account. Interestingly, enough, no one has ever been able to trace one cent of Hitler's considerable personal fortune, which he had received from the sale of his books and other income. Unlike his opponent, Franklin D. Roosevelt, Hitler had no trust fund from his mother (the proceeds from the China opium trade).

Dulles, as an international spymaster, would probably have been aware of Dr. Hoffmann's experiments. After he had returned to the United States and became director of the newly created CIA, Dulles ordered 10 kg of LSD from Sandoz, the stated purpose being "for use in drug experiments with animals and human beings. As there are some 10,000 doses per gram, this meant that Dulles ordered one hundred million doses of LSD. Meanwhile, a Dr. Timothy Leary had been hired by the National Institute of Health to experiment with psychedelic drugs, including LSD. Leary had already been forced to resign from West Point, and was later fired from the faculty at Harvard, perhaps the only person who could say this. Leary's NIH study was financed by a grant from the Uris Foundation of New York City. It continued from 1953 to 1956, when it was moved to the U.S. Public Health Service, the experiments going on until 1958, and also at HEW from 1956 to 1963. A CIA Memo dated November 1, 1963 featured glowing accounts of the work of Dr. Leary and his associate, Dr. Richard Alpert (who also was later fired from the staff at Harvard). They invented the turn on, tune in, drop out movement which incapacitated the youth of America for an entire generation. The movement, in which the CIA always had a proprietary interest, was given academic status when it was launched from the ivy-covered halls of Harvard by Leary and his group. After their forced departure from Harvard, they were esconced in a million dollar estate in New York by the wealthy Mellon heir, Tommy Hitchcock. Their movement swept over the campuses of American universities and destroyed the educational opportunities for thousands of American youths.

A later governmental investigation of the CIA, which was chaired, naturally enough, by Nelson Rockefeller, made this comment in its Rockefeller Report to the President on CIA activities, "Beginning in the late 1940s, the CIA began to study the properties of certain behaviour-influencing drugs ... all the records concerning the program were ordered destroyed in 1973, including a total of 152 separate files. CIA also contracted with the then Bureau of Narcotics to have mind-influencing drugs given to unwitting subjects in 'normal life-settings.' "

The above referred to several unfortunate incidents, in which CIA employees, who had been given doses of LSD without their knowledge, committed suicide under its malign influence. The families of these victims learned many years later of the true circumstances of these "suicides" and successfully sued the government to obtain financial settlements.

Of the various CIA projects, the most notorious was MK Ultra. These programs were supervised by another prototype of the "mad doctor," a Dr. Sidney Gottlieb. Despite the havoc wrought by his activities, Dr. Gottlieb was never brought to trial. Indeed, the then director of the CIA, Richard Helms, made certain that all records of the MK Ultra operation were destroyed during his last days in office, leaving Dr. Gottlieb immune to prosecution.

Dr. Gottleib, who has been described by observers as "a pharmaceutical Dr. Strangelove," envisioned dosing entire populations with hallucinogenic drugs. Influenced by his CIA experiments, the U.S. Army contemplated a program of driving whole populations insane with these drugs. Some 1,500 military personnel were then given LSD in tests run by the Army Chemical Corps, during the mid 1960s. Many of them suffered severe psychological damage, the most terrifying symptoms appearing years later. The Army then moved on to testing a more powerful chemical hallucinogen, which it called B.Z This drug was tested at Edgewood Arsenal between 1959 and 1975. About 2,800 soldiers were exposed to B.Z. Some of them have since lodged complaints that they suffered irreparable damage from the experiment.

One of the peripheral results of the CIA drug program was the assassination of President John F. Kennedy, the blame subsequently being laid at the door of various groups, the CIA, the Mafia, the Cuban Communists and others. The basis for these charges was that all of them were deeply involved. To cover up the trail, some forty people later died by violence. Some of them were media writers, the most prominent being the late Dorothy Kilgallen, a widely known columnist. In 1965 she used her connections to get permission to interview Jack Ruby in his prison cell. She later told friends that she had been able to obtain evidence that would "blow the J. F. Kennedy case sky high." Shortly afterwards, she was found in her apartment, dead of what was later diagnosed as an "overdose" of barbiturates and alcohol. The apartment was a shambles, and all of her notes of her conversations with Ruby had disappeared. To this day, no one has ever admitted seeing them. The Medical

Monopoly then used Kilgallen's death as an excuse to issue pious warning about "the dangers of mixing barbiturates and alcohol" but said nothing about the dangers of visiting Jack Ruby. Early in 1967, Ruby repeatedly complained that he was being poisoned. He was then diagnosed as having cancer, but he died of a "stroke," as did one of his accomplices, David Ferrie.

The apparition of Dr. Sidney Gottlieb as the CIA's "mad scientist" is eclipsed by the record of Dr. D. Ewen Cameron, who epitomized the Hollywood version of the insane doctor experimenting on helpless human subjects. Born in Scotland, Dr. Cameron moved to the United States, where he became a citizen. Although he carried on most of his medical work in Canada, he was a resident of Lake Placid, New York. The basis for the two-country operation may have been a desire to avoid lawsuits. In 1943, Dr. Cameron received a grant from the Rockefeller Foundation to set up a new psychiatric institute, the Allen Memorial Institute, as a wing of the Royal Victorian Hospital, the teaching hospital of McGill University in Montreal. This Rockefeller connection later resulted in some $10 million of CIA money being channelled to Cameron through Dr. Gottlieb as part of the MK Ultra project. This money was transferred to Dr. Cameron, beginning in 1953, because he had already demonstrated his commitment to mind-altering experiments. The CIA funds were therefore marked for mind control.

Dr. Cameron had come to the favorable attention of the Rockefeller interests after he invented some of the most terrifying "psychiatric" techniques ever known. He invented a process called "depatterning" as well as a later technique called "psychic driving," either of which would have done credit to any Communist brain washing expert. "Depatterning" began with heavy drug dosages, combined with electric shock, the then popular Electro Convulsive Therapy, or ECT, as it was usually known. It was later discredited for years because of the damage to the patients, but, incredibly, has now been revived and is in constant use in some circles. ECT has been described by its victims as the most terrifying ordeal which can be imagined. Basically, it was simply the electrocution process which was shut off just before it became fatal. The patient was strapped into a chair and electrocuted two or three times a day.

Initially, depatterning was limited to the heavy drug dosages, over a period from fifteen to thirty days; this part of the program was called "sleep therapy." A "sleep cocktail," which itself was worthy of the imagination of a Dr. Frankenstein, consisted of 100 mg of Thorazine, 100 mg of Nembutal, 100 mg of Seconal, 150 mg of Vernonal and 100 mg. of Phenergan, any one of which would be enough to put any patient to sleep. The sleep cocktail was administered to the patient three times a day. Later in the sleep therapy treatment, the patient was awakened two or three times a day to receive the electric shock treatments. Dr. Cameron ignored the recommended voltage for shock treatments, increasing them twenty to forty times higher than any other doctor had ever dared. He watched approvingly as the helpless patients screamed constantly during the electro-shock "therapy." It was his fond belief that the screams also were an essential part of the treatment, although it is likely that it represented his personal gratification.

The next step in depatterning, which was also one of the weirder Cameron inventions, was "sensory isolation," in which the patient was placed in a large box, with his eyes padded and his ears plugged. After some thirty days of the Cameron depatterning treatment, the patient was reduced to a helpless zombie. Satisfied that he had purged the patient of all previous images and ideas, Dr. Cameron moved into the next phase, which he called "psychic driving." This consisted of forcing the patient to listen to tape- recorded messages, repeated over and over, thousands of times. This "treatment" was administered through pillow speakers or headphones. Every intelligence agency in the world was green with envy when they heard of the new Cameron techniques. Luckily, the CIA had been the first on the scene, and provided him with ample funds for his lunatic obsessions.

Born in 1901 near Glasgow, Cameron had studied at the University of London, where he may have picked up some of his strange ideas. It is also likely that he became involved with some cult in London, which featured such monstrous ideas. After all, Mary Shelley had written Frankenstein in that very milieu.

Throughout his activities in Canada, the CIA Technical Services and the Staff Chemical Division enthusiastically funded his work.

Honors poured in on him, as word spread about his "innovative" techniques. He became chairman of the Canadian Psychiatric Association, chairman of the American Psychiatric Association, and founding chairman of the World Psychiatric Association.

After Dr. Cameron's death in 1967, the CIA found itself besieged by some of the survivors of his victims. In the most advanced stages of MK Ultra, he had experimented on some 53 people. This group included some prominent Canadians. An action was finally brought by Harry Weinstein, whose father Louis had been a leading Montreal businessman. Another victim was Velma Orlikon, wife of a Democratic Party Member of the Canadian Parliament. Despite these pedigrees, the victims found themselves up against a stone wall. The *Washington Post* noted in January, 1988, that the CIA was still fighting the action of nine elderly Canadians who had been drugged during the 1950s and who were asking $175,000 each in damages, later increased to $1,000,000 each. The case was then ordered to trial, after nine years of delaying tactics by the CIA, but no one is predicting a speedy solution.

During the Cameron era, the CIA continued its own experiments in the United States. They enlisted the services of a narcotic operator, George Hunter White, and set him up in an apartment in Greenwich Village. He was given a cover identity as an artist and a seaman, who met people at parties or in bars and lured them back to the apartment. The CIA money had transformed the seedy apartment into an espionage apparatus complete with two- way mirrors, surveillance and recording equipment and other tools of the trade. White dosed his visitors with LSD, while the CIA equipment meticulously recorded their reactions. These frequently consisted of "bad trips" in which the victims went temporarily insane, tried to commit suicide or murder and gave other evidences of the "mind control" which the CIA wished to learn.

To avoid exposure from complainants, the CIA transferred White to San Francisco, where he was given the run of two more CIA pads. He then initiated Operation Midnight Climax. Drug addicted prostitutes were paid to pick men up in local bars and bring them back for an orgy which featured drinks heavily laced with LSD. The ensuing action was taped and photographed in every detail, although the results are not likely to be made available to the Library of Congress.

Despite the excesses to which doctors such as Dr. Cameron and Dr. Sims went in their scientific enthusiasm, there are horror stories equally disturbing from the clinical experiments conducted by the ethical drug companies. With hundreds of millions in dollars of potential profits riding on each new drug product, the Medical Monopoly must comply with the regulations which they themselves have drafted and put into place. The purpose of the regulations is to protect the market share of a new wonder drug until it can be replaced by a newer wonder drug. As one alternative health care practitioner, who had been sent to prison for selling herbal teas, remarked, "A wonder drug is a drug that you take and then you wonder what it's going to do to you."

The restrictions on new drugs are usually complied with if the manufacturer believes it may be a big money maker. He is not about to release a new drug to the market, have it meet with success and then be forced to recall it because he has not complied with all of the regulations. From 1948 to 1958, pharmaceutical companies introduced 4,829 new products, 3,686 new compounds and 1,143 new dosages. All of these products had to go through the process.

New drugs are reported to take an average time of from seven to ten years to receive final FDA approval, a process which costs from ten to twelve million dollars, frequently as much as eighteen to twenty million. Clinical testing goes through three clearly defined phases. Phase I calls for the testing of the new drug on a small number of healthy people. Phase II requires that "volunteers" take the drug during a two year trial basis. Phase III calls for more diverse clinical testing on from one thousand to three thousand patients over a three year period. This means that doctors and hospitals administer the drug only because the Phase II testing has established its toxicity and other possible side effects. These are generally patients who are in a position to sue or generate unfavorable publicity if the drug proves to be dangerous, which means that those who prescribe the drug are relying on the Phase II testing to recommend it as reliable.

Phase II, in which the drug is tested on human beings, generally requires a captive population. The drugs are sometimes tested secretly in schools, hospitals and mental institutions, but the pharmaceutical manufacturers usually prefer to rely on a much safer test population, those confined to our prisons, because they are unlikely to complain. Even inmates of mental institutions have been known to complain, after their release, that they were subjected to illegal drug testing. Prisoners who have been convicted of crimes are less likely to complain. Since the turn of the century, the United States has led the world in the number of medical experiments carried on in prisons.

The law-abiding citizen might think that it is all right to conduct medical experiments on prisoners, even though a number of German doctors were executed for just such an offense. Drug testing might be one way in which the prisoner could repay his debt to society. However, the reality of the situation today is that, although there are many criminals confined in our prisons, there are also increasing numbers of Americans sent to prisons for political offenses. These political prisoners run the same risks in medical experiments as do the most hardened criminals. Each year, a larger number of sentences are handed down by American courts as punishment for banking problems, mortgage problems or tax problems.

Because of the Medical Monopoly's control of the media, the use of prisoners in medical experiments rarely comes to the attention of the American people. An exhaustive search of magazine indexes from 1900 to the present day reveals only a few such stories, which were uniformly favorable to the experiments. The prisoners themselves have little media access, unless they riot and bring the cameramen in in force, with the full top story treatment.

The American Medical Association is still the leading advocate of using prisoners for drug testing. The columnist, Pertinax, writing in the *British Medical Journal,* January 1963 commented, "I'm disturbed that the World Medical Association is now hedging on its clause about using criminals as experimental material. The AMA influence has been at work on its suspension. At the tenth meeting, American scientists joked about it. One of the nicest American scientists I know was heard to say 'Criminals in our prisons are fine experimental material—and much cheaper than chimpanzees'."

The scientist was not making a bad joke—chimpanzees cost as much as $4500 each, while American prisoners can be had for as little as one dollar a day. Pertinax was commenting on the proposal made by the World Medical Association in 1961, and offered for adoption, that "prisoners, being captive groups, should not be used as the subjects of experiments." The proposal was vociferously objected to by delegates from the American Medical Association and it was finally tabled.

If this smacks somewhat of the crimes of "Nazi doctors" and their experiments on prisoners, the coincidence is not accidental. The accused physicians testified in their own defense that they were merely following practices of long standing in the United States. At one trial, in 1947, 515 German doctors were tried at Nuremberg, indicted on the charge that they had conducted experiments on prisoners. They entered evidence in their defense that in 1906, American doctors in Philadelphia had used convicts for medical experiments, injecting them with plague and beri beri germs; in 1915, pellagra was injected into convicts in Massachusetts; in 1944, hundreds of prisoners in the United States were injected with malaria under the excuse of wartime necessity, to aid our soldiers in the Pacific. Despite this defense, the German doctors were convicted and some of them were executed.

The subject surfaced again with the recent publication of Robert Jay Lufton's book, "Nazi Doctors," one of the series of books about Nazis which pour from American presses in an ever- increasing stream, obeying the dictum that anything sells in the United States if a swastika is emblazoned on the cover. The book resulted in a spirited discussion in the Letters page of the *New York Times Sunday Book Review*. Bruno Bettelheim had originally reviewed the book, asserting that the effort to understand the Nazi doctors was wrong, "because of the ever-present danger that understanding fully may come close to forgiving." Christians, of course, offer forgiveness as a basic religious precept. Paul Ramsey wrote to include an excerpt from an advertisement, "Professor McCance and the members of the Medical Research Department want to be informed, if and when children are born in lying-in homes and women's wards in hospitals afflicted with Meningocele or similar abnormalities, which will make it unlikely that the children will survive longer than a short time. Professor McCance and his department wish to make some experiments on these children, which will give them no sorts of pains, but they feel not entitled to make these experiments on normal, healthy children.

When the birth of these children comes to be known, Professor McCance is to be informed at once by telephone."

Mr. Ramsey noted that this advertisement appeared in an American publication in 1946, while the German doctors were on trial. Telford Taylor, the American prosecutor at the Nuremberg trials, wrote to the *Times* to correct errors which had already appeared, including the statement that one of those sentenced was "Edwin Katzenellenbogen, who at one time had been a member of the faculty at Harvard Medical School." Taylor stated that no one by the name of Kazenellenbogen had ever been tried at Nuremberg.

Indeed, the name seems to have been included as an elaborate practical joke, the name having surfaced in previous practical jokes. The *Times* made no apology. Telford Taylor further pointed out that twenty physicians had been tried at Nuremberg in the instance mentioned, not nineteen as stated in the review, and that four were hanged, five sentenced to life in prison, three received lesser sentences and seven were acquitted on all charges."

Large scale medical experimentation, similar to that which was condemned as a crime at Nuremberg at the same time that it was still being practiced in American prisons, takes undue advantage of the "volunteers." Some are illiterate; most are young and healthy and have never had any serious illness. They have little concept of what it may be like to come down with a serious illness as a result of being injected with experimental drugs, or the lifelong complications which may result.

In 1963, *Time* magazine ran an expose of large scale programs which federal government officials had established in our prisons. These vast testing programs were justified as being part of the "war on cancer" which Bobst and the Laskers had launched from the White House. The doctors were injecting prisoners with live cancer cells and with blood from persons suffering from leukemia. Several doctors in Oklahoma were grossing three hundred thousand dollars a year from drug manufacturers in these deals; these doctors also regularly collected blood from prisoners, paying them $7 a quart; they then sold the blood for $15.

During the 1940s, when the first stories about the use of prisoners in medical experiments began to receive some circulation, the American Medical Association requested Governor Dwight of Illinois to scotch the stories. He whitewashed the experiments by appointing Morris Fishbein and other AMA leaders to a committee which solemnly "investigated" the programs and returned with glowing reports. Fishbein himself came back from Stateville Penitentiary to describe the prisoner experiments as "ideal, because of their conformity with ethical rules." Fishbein elaborated his enthusiasm by pointing out that the program rendered a genuine service to the entire public because of the "reformation value in serving as a subject in a medical experiment." One might have expected Fishbein to appear at Nuremberg, to defend the German doctors with the same argument, that they had offered this same "reformation value" to the inmates of the concentration camps. A public relations spokesman for Wyeth laboratories was puzzled by the indignation in some quarters, releasing a statement that "Almost all of our Phase II testing is done on prisoners."

In fact, there was fierce and ongoing competition among the major drug firms to line up prisoners who could be used as "subjects" in medical experiments. Upjohn and Parke-Davis adhered to established principles of monopoly when they acquired "exclusive rights" to the inmates of Jackson State Prison in Mississippi. These firms subsequently were able to enroll 1,200 of the 4,000 convicts there in the testing program. *Business Week* offered a somewhat critical comment on the program, pointing out that "tests at the prison are designed primarily to measure the toxicity of the drug rather than its efficiency. doses are built up gradually to the point where adverse reactions occur." In plainer English, the dosage was increased until it made the prisoner so ill or caused serious damage. The results often were crippling or death.

However, the prisoners were paid thirty cents a day for submitting to these experiments. *Business Week* touched upon the fact that it was precisely the life-threatening aspect of Phase II testing for which the prisoners were needed. The pharmaceutical companies needed to know how many people might be injured by the drug, or how many lawsuits they might expect from angry customers.

The drug testing programs were welcomed by prison officials, who maintained ancient buildings dating back to the Civil War to house the prisoners, while they built themselves monumental new administration offices and other perquisites of the trade. In 1971, the New York State Prison System spent $5,500 a year for each prisoner in the system, of which 72 cents a day went for food, and 15 cents a day for clothing and other amenities. Of the budgeted $17 a day per prisoner, less than a dollar a day went for his physical maintenance. This was an essential part of a prison system which had been set up the Boss Tweed and which still offered many golden opportunities to those who were alert.

Only a few stories leaked out to the public during these postwar years. Prisons are closed systems and investigative reporters are rarely welcomed. One of the most horrifying, which would have shamed any Nazi doctor, came from Vacaville State Prison in California. Extensive testing programs had been carried out here for years. A few of the prisoners were paid $15 a month, but most of them received only a dollar a day. The victims reported an alarming list of results, such as heart damage, loss of hair, joint pains, swelling of the legs, shortness of breath and hemorrhages of the skin. One testing outfit, under the name of the Solano Institute for Medical and Physical Research, actually was able to set up its headquarters at the prison. Established as a nonprofit corporation under the California charitable trust law, the "Institute" subjected 1,500 prisoners to various types of injections. One prisoner who had been sent to Vacaville for "treatment" later sued the doctor, a leading dermatologist who was head of his professional association. The prisoner had been forced to take muscular injections of Lederle's Caridase drug. This drug contained fibrinolytic enzymes which were intended for use as an anti-inflammatory agent. The patient testified that he had been seized by trustees and held while he was forcibly injected in both arms. He subsequently developed a near-fatal disease of the muscles and chronic stomach ulcers, while his weight dropped from 140 pounds to a mere 75 pounds. He received four dollars in compensation.

The King of the Prison Experiments was one Dr. Austin Stough. He had initiated contracts with the nation's largest pharmaceutical manufacturers to carry out drug testing at a number of prisons in three southern states, Alabama, Arkansas and Oklahoma. The program, to test blood plasma, at its peak involved 137 prisons from 1963 to 1970 and was paid for by 37 drug companies, including such leading firms as Upjohn, Wyeth, Lederle, Squibb and Merck. Although the financial rewards were impressive, the results of the program proved inconclusive. The program was later criticized as operating under "gross mismanagement, sloppy handling and contamination" of test samples, criticism which put an end to the program. Hundreds of prisoners suffered from its after effects for years. Stough had set up a prison monopoly which brought in good returns until his methods were exposed as being worthless.

Despite the dramatic implications of the drug testing stories, they met with thunderous silence from the "bleeding hearts" of the nation's media, perhaps because publicity about these programs might have raised conjecture as to why German doctors had been executed for the same practices. A survey of *Readers Guide,* the index to magazine articles printed throughout the United States, showed that from 1945 to 1970, during the height of the testing programs in the prisons, there were only three stories about it during this entire period. The first, a heart warming story in *Coronet,* November 1950, was titled "Prison Heroes Conquer Malaria," a glowing account of experiments conducted at the Illinois State Prison at Joliet, where Dr. Fishbein himself had been overwhelmed by the "ethical" nature of the drug testing program. The second story, in the *Saturday Evening Post,* March 2, 1963, was titled "Convict Volunteers." It too was an uncritical account of the drug experimenters, describing the prisoners as "human guinea pigs." The journalist quoted one convict, who was deliberately burned on both arms, "The pain was pretty bad," and mentioned other prisoners who had been injected with live cancer cells. Despite the fact that this story, written about inmates at the Ohio State Prison in Columbus, mentioned that these convicts did not receive any pay for submitting to these experiments (Ohio statutes piously forbid such payments, saving the drug companies even more money), the writer ends his article with a glowing tribute to the program, pointing out that it caused "the volunteers to feel self-respect."

The third story, in *Business Week,* June 27, 1964, noted that the drug companies were able to save many millions of dollars by using the prisoners for drug experiments.

CHAPTER 10

THE ROCKEFELLER SYNDICATE

Many American conservatives believe as a matter of faith that the Rockefellers and the Council on Foreign Relations exercise absolute control over the government and the people of United States. This thesis can be accepted as a working formula if one remains conscious of the larger issues. Two writers for whom the present writer has great respect, Dr. Emanuel Josephson and Morris Bealle, insisted on focusing on the Rockefellers and excluding all other aspects of the World Order. This severely limited the effect of their otherwise groundbreaking work on the Medical Monopoly.

This writer advanced a contrary view in *"The World Order,"*[3] fixing upon the Rothschild monetary power, which reached a point of world control by 1885, and its London policy group, the Royal Institute of International Affairs, as the policy makers for what has essentially been since 1900, a re-established colonial government in the United States. The colonial, or occupation, government, functions primarily through the Council on Foreign Relations, but only as the subsidiary of RIIA and through the Rockefeller Foundation, which controls government functions, the educational establishments, the media, the religions and the state legislatures.

---

[3] Published by Omnia Veritas Ltd.

It is true that the American colonials have "free elections," in which they have the absolute right to vote for one of two opposing candidates, both of whom have been handpicked and financed by the Rockefeller syndicate. This touching evidence of "democracy" serves to convince most Americans that we are indeed a free people. We even have a cracked Liberty Bell in Philadelphia to prove it.

American youths have been free since 1900 to be marched off to die in Hegelian wars in which both combatants received their instructions from the World Order. We are free to invest in a stock market in which the daily quantity, price and value of the monetary unit is manipulated and controlled by a Federal Reserve System which is answerable only to the Bank of England. It has maintained its vaunted "independence" from our government control, but this is the only independence it has ever had.

The realization that we do indeed live under the dictates of the "Rockefeller Syndicate" can well be the starting point of the long road back of a genuine struggle for American independence. In exposing "the Rockefellers" as agents of a foreign power, which is not merely a foreign power, but a genuine world government, we must realize that this is not merely a group dedicated to making money, but a group which is committed to maintaining the power of a colonial form of government over the American people. Thus the ancient calumny of John D. Rockefeller as a man obsessed by greed (a category in which he has plenty of company) obscures the fact that from the day the Rothschilds began to finance his march towards a total oil monopoly in the United States from their coffers at the National City Bank of Cleveland, Rockefeller was never an independent power, nor does any department of the Rockefeller Syndicate operate as an independent power. We know that the Cosa Nostra, or Mafia, with which the Syndicate is closely allied has somewhat autonomous power in the regions which have been assigned to that particular "family" by the national directors, but this always implies that that family remains under total control and answerable for everything which occurs in its territory.

Similarly, the Rockefeller Syndicate operates under clearly defined spheres of influence. The "charitable" organizations, the business companies and the policy groups, always meld into a working operation, nor can any department of the Syndicate strike out on its own or formulate an independent policy, no matter what may be its justification.

The Rockefeller Syndicate operates under the control of the world financial structure, which means that on any given day, all of its assets could be rendered close to worthless by adroit financial manipulation. This is the the final control, which ensures that no one can quit the organization. Not only would he be stripped of all assets, but he would be under contract for immediate assassination. Our Department of Justice is well aware that the only "terrorists" operating in the United States are the agents of the World Order, but they prudently avoid any mention of this fact.

The world financial structure, far from being an unknown or hidden organization, is actually well known and well defined. It consists of the major Swiss Banks; the survivors of the old Venetian-Genoese banking axis; the Big Five of the world grain trade; the British combine, centered in the Bank of England and its chartered merchant banks, functioning through the Rothschilds and the Oppenheimers and having absolute control over their Canadian colony through the Royal Bank of Canada and the Bank of Montreal, their Canadian lieutenants being the Bronfmans, Belzbergs, Reichmanns and other financial operators; and the colonial banking structure in the United States, controlled by the Bank of England through the Federal

Reserve System; the Boston Brahmin families who made their fortunes in the opium trade, including the Delanos and others and the Rockefeller Syndicate, consisting of the Kissinger network headquartered in the Rockefeller Bank, Chase Manhattan Bank, American Express, the present form of the old Rothschild representatives in the United States, which includes Kuhn, Loeb Company and Lehman Brothers. It is notable that the Rockefeller Syndicate is far down on the list of the world's financial structure. Why then is it of such importance? Although it is not the crucial factor in financial decision in the Western Hemisphere, it is the actual working control mechanism of the American colony. The Rockefeller family themselves, like the Morgans, Schiffs and Warburgs, have faded into insignificance, but the mechanism created in their name roars along at full power, still maintaining all of the functions for which it was organized. Since he set up the Trilateral Commission, David Rockefeller has functioned as a sort of international courier for the World Order, principally concerned with delivering working instructions to the Communist bloc, either directly, in New York or by travelling to the area.

Laurance Rockefeller is active in the operation of the Medical Monopoly, but his principal interests are in operating various vacation spas in tropical areas. They are the two survivors of the "Fortunate Five," the five sons of John D. Rockefeller, Jr. and Abby Aldrich. John D. Rockefeller, Jr. died in an institution in Tucson, Arizona and was hastily cremated. John D. Rockefeller III died in a mysterious accident on a New York Parkway near his home. Nelson Rockefeller, named after his grandfather, died in the arms of a TV journalist; it was later revealed that he had also been in the arms of another TV journalist at the same time; the death was hushed up for many hours. It is generally believed that he ran afoul of his Colombian drug connection, the disagreement hardly being trivial; it involved several billion dollars in drug profits which had not been properly apportioned. Winthrop Rockefeller died an alcoholic in the arms of his black boy friend. He had been interviewed on television by Harry Reasoner to explain his hasty move from New York to Arkansas. Winthrop leered that his black boy friend, an Army sergeant who apparently taught him the mysteries of drill, refused to live in New York. To celebrate this alliance, Winthrop Rockefeller gave magnificently to Negro causes, including the Urban League building on East 48th Street in New York. A plaque on the second floor notes that it was his gift; it might well have stated "From Hadrian to his Anti-nous."

We do not wish to imply that the Rockefellers no longer have influence, but that the major policy dictates of the Rockefeller Syndicate are handed down by other capos, of whom they continue to be a visible force. Through the person of David Rockefeller, the family is sometimes called "the first family of the Soviet Union." Only he and Dr. Armand Hammer, the moving force behind USTEC, have permanent permission to land their private planes at the Moscow Airport. Others would suffer the fate of KAL 007.

David Rockefeller's most significant trip to the Soviet Union may have been the fateful day when he landed in Moscow, having been told to inform Khrushchev that he was "through." The Russians are very health conscious, and a scientist had sent information to Khrushchev that the use of chemical fertilizers in the Soviet Union presented a threat to the people. Khrushchev then announced a major change in the Soviet farm policy, centering around a reduction in the use of chemicals. This was upsetting to the head of the world's Chemical Fertilizer Trust, David Rockefeller, and he responded with a terse one word command, "Out."

Both the Rockefeller family fortune and the considerable portion set aside in the foundations of the Rockefeller

Syndicate are effectively insulated against any type of government control.

Fortune magazine noted August 4, 1986, that John D. Rockefeller, Jr. had created trusts in 1934 which now amounted to some $2.3 billion; another $200 million had been set aside for the Abby Rockefeller branch. The five sons had trusts which in 1986 amount to $2.1 billion. These trusts had originally amounted to only $50 million each, showing the increase in their assets as well as inflation during the ensuing half century. *Fortune* estimated the 1986 total Rockefeller wealth as $3.5 billion, of which $900 million was in securities and real estate. They owned 45% of the Time Life Building; Nelson Rockefeller's International Basic Economy Corporation had been sold to a British company in 1980. For years, the Rockefeller family had deliberately kept the rents low in its major holding, Rockefeller Center, a $1.6 billion investment yielding an annual return of 1%. This was a convenient maneuver for tax purposes. Rockefeller Center recently went public, issuing stock which was sold to public buyers. The Rockefellers are rumored to be liquidating their investments in the New York area, and reinvesting in the West, particularly in the area around Phoenix, Arizona. It is possible that they know something we don't.

However much of the Rockefeller wealth may be attributed to old John D.'s rapacity and ruthlessness, its origins are indubitably based in his initial financing from the National City Bank of Cleveland, which was identified in Congressional reports as one of the three Rothschild banks in the United States and by his later acceptance of the guidance of Jacob Schiff of Kuhn, Loeb Company, who had been born in the Rothschild house in Frankfort and was now the principal Rothschild representative (but unknown as such to the public) in the United States.

With the seed money from the National City Bank of Cleveland, old John D. Rockefeller soon laid claim to the title of "the most ruthless American." It is more than likely that it was this quality which persuaded the Rothschilds to back him. Rockefeller realized early in the game that the oil refinery business, which could offer great profits in a short time, also was at the mercy of uncontrolled competition. His solution was a simple one—crush all competition. The famous Rockefeller dedication to total monopoly was simply a business decision. Rockefeller embarked on a campaign of coercing all competing oil refineries out of business.

He attacked on a number of fronts, which is also a lesson to all would be entrepreneurs. First, he would send a minion, not known to be working for Rockefeller, with an offer to buy the competing refinery for a low price, but offering cash. If the offer was refused, the competitor would then come under attack from a competing refinery which greatly undercut his price. He might also suffer a sudden strike at his refinery, which would force him to shut down. Control of labor through unions has always been a basic Rockefeller technique. Like the Soviet Union, they seldom have labor trouble. If these techniques failed, Rockefeller would then be saddened by a reluctant decision to use violence; beating the rival workers as they went to and from their jobs, or burning or blowing up the competing refinery.

These techniques convinced the Rothschilds that they had found their man. They sent their personal representative, Jacob Schiff, to Cleveland to help Rockefeller plan further expansion. At this time, the Rothschilds controlled 95% of all railroad mileage in the United States, through the J. P. Morgan Company and Kuhn Loeb Company according to official Department of Commerce figures for the year 1895. J. P. Morgan mentions in his *Who's Who* listing that he controlled 50,000 miles of U.S. railways. Schiff worked out an elaborate rebate deal for Rockefeller, through a dummy corporation, South Improvement Company. These rebates ensured that no other oil company could survive in competition with the Rockefeller firm. The scheme was later exposed, but by that time, Rockefeller had achieved a virtual monopoly of the oil business in the United States. The daughter of one of his victims, Ida Tarbell, whose father was ruined by Rockefeller's criminal operations, wrote the first major expose of the Standard Oil Trust.

She was promptly denounced as a "muckraker" by the poseur, Theodore Roosevelt, who claimed to be a "trustbuster." In fact, he ensured the dominance of the Standard Oil Trust and other giant trusts.

During the next half century, John D. Rockefeller was routinely caricatured by socialist propagandists as the epitome of the ruthless capitalist. At the same time, he was the principal financier of the world Communist movement, through a firm called American International Company. Despite the fact that the House of Rothschild had already achieved world control, the sound and fury was directed exclusively against its two principal, representatives, John D. Rockefeller and J. P. Morgan. One of the few revelations of the actual state of affairs appeared in *Truth* magazine, December 16, 1912, which pointed out that "Mr. Schiff is head of the great private banking house of Kuhn, Loeb Company, which represents the Rothschild interests on this side of the Atlantic. He is described as a financial strategist and has been for years the financial minister of the great impersonal power known as Standard Oil." Note that this editor did not even mention the name of Rockefeller.

Because of these concealed factors, it was a relatively simple matter for the American public to accept the "fact" that the Rockefellers were the preeminent power in this country. This myth was actually clothed in the apparel of power, the Rockefeller Oil Trust becoming the "military-industrial complex" which assumed political control of the nation; the Rockefeller Medical Monopoly attained control of the health care of the nation, and the Rockefeller Foundation, a web of affiliated tax exempt creations, effectively controlled the religious and educational life of the nation. The myth succeeded in its goal of camouflaging the hidden rulers, the Rothschilds.

After the present writer had been exposing this charade for some twenty-five years, a new myth began to be noised about in American conservative circles, effectively propagated by active double agents. This myth found a host of eager believers, because it heralded a growing crack in the monolithic power which had been oppressing all the peoples of the world. This new "revelation" was that a struggle to the death for world power had developed between the Rockefellers and the Rothschilds. According to this startling development, one faction or the other, depending on which agent you were listening to, had gained control of the Soviet Union and would use its power as the basis for achieving the overthrow of the other action. The sudden death of several members of the Rockefeller family was cited as "proof that such a struggle was taking place, although no Rothschild is known to have succumbed during this "war." This ignored the general understanding that Nelson Rockefeller had been "eliminated" as the result of losing deposit slips for several billion dollars of drugs from the Colombian cartel, or that the other Rockefeller deaths showed no trace of a "Rothschild connection."

Having maintained extensive files on this situation for several decades, the present writer could not believe anyone could be so misinformed as to think that "the Rockefellers" were now trying to seize power from the Rothschilds, at a time when the influence of members of the Rockefeller family was already in great decline, their family finances being handled by J. Richardson Dilworth, their legal affairs being handled by John J. McCloy, and other faithful retainers; none of these retainers would have been willing to engage in a genuine power struggle, as they were faceless managers who lived only for their weekly paycheck. They had no ambitions of their own. Nevertheless, many hopeful Americans grasped at the will-o-the-wisp notion that the Rockefellers were now "good Americans" who were willing to risk all to overthrow the Rothschilds. Amazingly enough, this pernicious story persisted for almost a decade before being relegated to the curiosities of history.

Like J. P. Morgan, who had begun his commercial career by selling the U.S. Army some defective guns, the famous Hall carbine affair, John D. Rockefeller also was a war profiteer during the Civil War; he sold unstamped Harkness liquor to Federal troops at a high profit, gaining the initial capital to embark on his drive for monopoly. His interest in the oil business was a natural one; his father, William Rockefeller had been "in oil" for years. William Rockefeller had become an oil entrepreneur after salt wells at Tarentum, near Pittsburgh, were discovered in 1842 to be flowing with oil. The owners of the wells, Samuel L. Kier, began to bottle the oil and sell it for medicinal purposes. One of his earliest wholesalers was William Rockefeller. The "medicine" was originally labelled "Kier's Magic Oil." Rockefeller printed his own labels, using "Rock Oil" or "Seneca Oil," Seneca being the name of a well known Indian tribe. Rockefeller achieved his greatest notoriety and his greatest profits by advertising himself as "William Rockefeller, the Celebrated Cancer Specialist." It is understandable that his grandsons would become the controlling power behind the scenes of the world's most famous cancer treatment center and would direct government funds and charitable contributions to those areas which only benefit the Medical Monopoly. William Rockefeller spared no claim in his flamboyant career. He guaranteed "All Cases of Cancer Cured Unless

They Are Too Far Gone." Such were the healing powers that he attributed to his magic cancer cure that he was able to retail it for $25 a bottle, a sum then equivalent to two months' wages. The "cure" consisted of a few well known diuretics, which had been diluted by water. This carnival medicine show barker could hardly have envisioned that his descendants would control the greatest and the most profitable Medical Monopoly in recorded history.

As an itinerant "carnie," a travelling carnival peddler, William Rockefeller had chosen a career which interfered with developing a stable family life. His son John rarely saw him, a circumstance which has inspired some psychological analysts to conjecture that the absence of a father figure or parental love may have contributed to John D. Rockefeller's subsequent development as a money mad tyrant who plotted to maim, poison and kill millions of his fellow American during almost a century of his monopolistic operations and whose influence, reaching up from the grave, remains the most dire and malignant presence in American life. This may have been a contributing factor—however, it is also possible that he was totally evil. It is hardly arguable that he is probably the most Satanic figure in American history.

It has long been a truism that you can find a horse thief or two in any prominent American family. In the Rockefeller family, it was more than a truism. William seems to have faithfully followed the precepts of the Will of Canaan throughout his career, "love robbery, love lechery." He fled from a number of indictments for horse stealing, finally disappearing altogether as William Rockefeller and re-emerging as a Dr. William Levingston of Philadelphia, a name which he retained for the rest of his life. An investigative reporter at Joseph Pulitzer's New York World received a tip that was followed up. The World then disclosed that William Avery Rockefeller had died May 11, 1906 in Freeport, Illinois, where he was interred in an

unmarked grave as Dr. William Levingston. William
Rockefeller's vocation as a medicine man greatly facilitated
his preferred profession of horse thief. As one who planned
to be in the next county by morning, it was a simple matter
to tie a handsome stallion to the back of his wagon and head
for the open road. It also played a large part in his vocation
as a woman-chaser; he was described as being "woman-
mad." He not only concluded several bigamous marriages,
but he seems to have had uncontrolled passions. On June
28, 1849, he was indicted for raping a hired girl in Cayuga,
New York; he later was found to be residing in Oswego,
New York and was forced once again to decamp for parts
unknown. He had no difficulty in financing his woman-
chasing interests from the sale of his miraculous cancer cure
and from another product, his "Wonder Working
Liniment," which he offered at only two dollars a bottle. It
consisted of crude petroleum from which the lighter oils had
been boiled away, leaving a heavy solution of paraffin, lube
oil and tar, which comprised the "liniment." William
Rockefeller's original miracle oil survived until quite recently
as a concoction called Nujol, consisting principally of
petroleum and peddled as a laxative. It was well known that
Nujol was merely an advertising sobriquet meaning "new
oil," as opposed, apparently, to "old oil." Sold as an antidote
to constipation, it robbed the body of fat-soluble vitamins, it
being a well-established medical fact that mineral oil coated
the intestine and prevented the absorption of many needed
vitamins and other nutritional needs. Its makers added
carotene as a sop to the health-conscious, but it was hardly
worth the bother. Nujol was manufactured by a subsidiary
of Standard Oil of New Jersey, called Stanco, whose only
other product, manufactured on the same premises, was the
famous insecticide, Flit.

Nujol was hawked from the Senate Office Building in
Washington for years during a more liberal interpretation of
"conflict of interest." In this case, it was hardly a conflict of

interest, because the august peddler, Senator Royal S. Copeland, never had any interests other than serving the Rockefellers. He was a physician whom Rockefeller had appointed as head of the New York State Department of Health and later financed his campaign for the Senate. Copeland's frank display of commercialism amazed even the most blase Washington reporters. He devoted his Senate career to a daily program advertising Nujol. A microphone was set up in his Senate office each morning, the first order of business being the Nujol program, for which he was paid $75,000 a year, an enormous salary in the 1930s and more than the salary of the President of the United States. Senator Copeland's exploits earned him a number of nicknames on Capitol Hill. He was often called the Senator from the American Medical Association, because of his enthusiastic backing for any program launched by the AMA and Morris Fishbein. More realistically, he was usually referred to as "the Senator from Standard Oil." He could be counted on to promote any legislation devised for the greater profit of the Rockefeller monopoly. During congressional debate on the Food and Drug Act in 1938, he came under criticism from Congresswoman Leonor Sullivan, who charged that Senator Copeland, a physician who handled the bill on the Senate floor, frankly acknowledged during the debate that soap was exempted from the law, because the soap manufacturers, who were the nation's largest advertisers, would otherwise join with other big industries to fight the bill. Congressman Sullivan complained the "Soap was officially declared in the law not to be a cosmetic. The hair dye manufacturers were given a license to market known dangerous products, just so long as they placed a special warning on the label—but what woman in a beauty parlor ever sees the label on the bulk container in which hair dye is shipped?"

Just as the elder Rockefeller had spent his life in the pursuit of his personal obsession, women, so his son John was equally obsessed, being money-mad instead of women-mad, totally committed to the pursuit of ever-increasing wealth and power.

However, the principal accomplishments of the Rockefeller drive for power, the rebate scheme for monopoly, the chartering of the foundations to gain power over American citizens, the creation of the central bank, the Federal Reserve System, the backing of the World Communist revolution and the creation of the Medical Monopoly, all came from the Rothschilds or from their European employees. We cannot find in the records of John D. Rockefeller that he originated any one of these programs. The concept of the tax exempt charitable foundation originated with the Rothschild minion, George Pea-body, in 1865. The Peabody Educational Foundation later became the Rockefeller Foundation. It is unlikely that even the diabolical mind of John D. Rockefeller could have conceived of this devious twist. A social historian has described the major development of the late nineteenth century, when charitable foundations and world Communism became important movements, as one of the more interesting facets of history, perhaps equivalent to the discovery of the wheel. This new discovery was the concept developed by the rats, who after all have rather highly developed intelligences, that they could trap people by baiting traps with little bits of cheese. The history of mankind since then has been the rats catching humans in their traps. Socialism—indeed, any government program—is simply the rat baiting the trap with a smidgeon of cheese and catching himself a human.

Congressman Wright Putman, chairman of the House Banking and Currency Committee, noted from the floor of Congress that the establishment of the Rockefeller Foundation effectively insulated Standard Oil from competition. The controlling stock had been removed from market manipulation or possible buyouts by competitors. It also relieved Standard Oil from most taxation, which then placed a tremendous added burden on individual American taxpayers. Although a Rockefeller relative by marriage, Senator Nelson Aldrich, Republican majority leader in the Senate, had pushed the General Education Board charter through Congress, the Rockefeller Foundation charter proved to be more difficult.

Widespread criticism of Rockefeller's monopolistic practices was heard, and his effort to insulate his profits from taxation or takeover was seen for what it was. The charter was finally pushed through in 1913 (the significant Masonic numeral 13—1913 was also the year of the progressive income tax and of the enactment of the Federal Reserve Act). Senator Robert F. Wagner of New York, another Senator from Standard Oil (there were quite a few), ramrodded the Congressional approval of the charter. The charter was then signed by John D. Rockefeller, John D. Rockefeller, Jr., Henry Pratt Judson, president of the Rockefeller established University of Chicago, Simon Flexner, director of the Rockefeller Institute, Starr Jameson, described in *Who's Who* as "personal counsel to John D. Rockefeller in his benevolences," and Charles W. Eliot, president of Harvard University.

The Rockefeller Oil Monopoly is now 125 years old, yet in 1911, the Supreme Court, bowing to public outrage, had ruled that it had to be broken up. The resulting companies proved to be no problem for the Rockefeller interests. The family retained a two per cent holding in each of the "new" companies, while the Rockefeller foundations took a three per cent stock holding in each company.

This gave them a five per cent stock interest in each company; a one per cent holding in a corporation is usually sufficient to maintain working control.

The involvement of the Rockefellers in promoting the world Communist Revolution also developed from their business interests. There was never any commitment to the Marxist ideology; like anything else, it was there to be used. At the turn of the century, Standard Oil was competing fiercely with Royal Dutch Shell for control of the lucrative European market. Congressional testimony revealed that Rockefeller had sent large sums to Lenin and Trotsky to instigate the Communist Revolution of 1905. His banker, Jacob Schiff, had previously financed the Japanese in their war against Russia and had sent a personal emissary, George Kennan to Russia to spend some twenty years in promoting revolutionary activity against the Czar. When the 1905 revolution failed, Lenin was placed "in storage" in Switzerland until 1917. Trotsky was brought to the United States, where he lived rent free on the Standard Oil property at Bayonne, New Jersey, its tank field. When the Czar abdicated, Trotsky was placed on a ship with three hundred Communist revolutionaries from the Lower East Side of New York. Rockefeller obtained a special passport for Trotsky from Woodrow Wilson and sent Lincoln Steffens with him to make sure he was returned safely to Russia. For traveling expenses, Rockefeller placed a purse containing $10,000 in Trotsky's pocket.

On April 13, 1917, when the ship stopped in Halifax, Canadian Secret Service officers immediately arrested Trotsky and interred him in Nova Scotia. The case became an international cause celebre, as leading government officials from several nations frantically demanded Trotsky's release. The Secret Service had been tipped off that Trotsky was on his way to take Russia out of the war, freeing more German armies to attack Canadian troops on the Western Front. Prime Minister Lloyd George hurriedly cabled orders from London to the Canadian Secret Service to free Trotsky at once— they ignored him. Trotsky was finally freed by the intervention of one of Rockefeller's most faithful stooges,

Canadian Minister Mackenzie King, who had long been a "labor specialist" for the Rockefellers. King personally obtained Trotsky's release and sent him on his way as the emissary of the Rockefellers, commissioned to win the Bolshevik Revolution. Thus Dr. Armand Hammer, who loudly proclaims his influence in Russia as the friend of Lenin, has an insignificant claim compared to the role of the Rockefellers in backing world Communism. Although Communism, like other isms, had originated with Marx's association with the House of Rothschild, it enlisted the reverent support of John D. Rockefeller because he saw Communism for what it is, the ultimate monopoly, not only controlling the government, the monetary system and all property, but also a monopoly which, like the corporations it emulates, is self-perpetuating and eternal. It was the logical progression from his Standard Oil monopoly.

An important step on the road to world monopoly was the most far-reaching corporation invented by the Rothschilds. This was the international drug and chemical cartel, I. G. Farben. Called "a state within a state," it was created in 1925 as Interessen Gemeinschaft Farbeindustrie Aktien gesellschaft, usually known as I. G. Farben, which simply meant "The Cartel." It had originated in 1904, when the six major chemical companies in Germany began negotiations to form the ultimate cartel, merging Badische Anilin, Bayer, Agfa, Hoechst, Weiler-ter-Meer, and Greisheim-Electron. The guiding spirit, as well as the financing, came from the Rothschilds, who were represented by their German banker, Max Warburg, of M. M. Warburg Company, Hamburg. He later headed the German Secret Service during World War I and was personal financial adviser to the Kaiser. When the Kaiser was overthrown, after losing the war, Max Warburg was not exiled with him to Holland; instead, he became the financial adviser to the new government. Monarchs may come and go, but the real power remains with the bankers. While representing

Germany at the Paris Peace Conference, Max Warburg spent pleasant hours renewing family ties with his brother, Paul Warburg, who, after drafting the Federal Reserve Act at Jekyl Island, had headed the U.S. banking system during the war. He was in Paris as Woodrow Wilson's financial advisor.

I. G. Farben soon had a net worth of six billion marks, controlling some five hundred firms. Its first president was Professor Carl Bosch. During the period of the Weimar Republic, I. G. officials, seeing the handwriting on the wall, began a close association with Adolf Hitler, supplying much needed funds and political influence. The success of the I. G. Farben cartel had aroused the interest of other industrialists. Henry Ford was favorably impressed and set up a German branch of Ford Motor Company. Forty per cent of the stock was purchased by I. G. Farben. I. G. Farben then established an American subsidiary, called American I. G., in cooperation with Standard Oil of New Jersey. Its directors included Walter Teagle, president of Standard Oil, Paul Warburg of Kuhn, Loeb Company and Edsel Ford, representing the Ford interests. John Foster Dulles, for the law firm, Sullivan and Cromwell, became the attorney for I. G., frequently travelling between New York and Berlin on cartel business. His law partner, Arthur Dean, is now director of the $40 million Teagle Foundation which was set up before Teagle's death. Like other fortunes, it had become part of the network. Like John Foster Dulles, Arthur Dean has been a director of American Banknote for many years; this is the firm which supplies the paper for our dollar bills. Dean also has been an active behind the scenes government negotiator, serving as arms negotiator at disarmament on conferences. Dean was also a director of Rockefeller's American Ag&Chem Company. He was a director of American Solvay, American Metal and other firms. As attorney for the wealthy Hochschild family, who owned Climax Molybdenum and American Metal, Dean became director of their family foundation, the Hochschild

Foundation. Dean is director emeritus of the Council on Foreign Relations, the Asia Foundation, International House, Carnegie Foundation, and the Sloan Kettering Cancer Center.

In 1930, Standard Oil announced that it had purchased an alcohol monopoly in Germany, a deal which had been set up by I. G. Farben. After Hitler came to power, John D. Rockefeller assigned his personal press agent, Ivy Lee, to Hitler to serve as a fulltime adviser on the rearmament of Germany, a necessary step for setting up World War EL Standard Oil then built large refineries in Germany for the Nazis and continued to supply them with oil during World War II. In the 1930s, Standard Oil was receiving in payment from Germany large shipments of musical instruments and ships which had been built in German yards.

The dreaded Gestapo, the Nazi police force, was actually built from the worldwide intelligence network which I. G. Farben had maintained since its inception. Herman Schmitz, who had succeeded Carl Bosch as head of I. G., has been personal advisor to chancellor Breuning; when Hitler took over, Schmitz then became his most trusted secret counselor. So well concealed was the association that the press had orders never to photograph them together. Schmitz was named an honorary member of the Reichstag, while his assistant, Carl Krauch, became Goering's principal advisor in carrying out the Nazis' Four Year Plan. A business associate, Richard Krebs, later testified before the House Un-American Activities Committee, "The I. G. Farbinindustrie, I know from personal experience, was already, in 1934, completely in the hands of the Gestapo." This was a misstatement; the I. G. Farben had merely allied itself with the Gestapo.

In 1924, Krupp Industries was in serious financial difficulty; the firm was saved by a $10 million cash loan from Hallgarten & Company and Goldman Sachs, two of Wall Street's best known firms. The planned re-armament of Germany was able to proceed only after Dillon Read floated $100 million of German bonds on Wall Street for that purpose. It was hardly surprising that at the conclusion of the Second World War, General William Draper was appointed Economic Czar of Germany, being named head of the Economic Division of the Allied Military Government. He was a partner of Dillon Read.

In 1939, Frank Howard, a vice-president of Standard Oil, visited Germany. He later testified, "We did our best to work out complete plans for a modus vivendi which would operate throughout the term of the war, whether we came in or not." At this time, American I. G. had on its board of directors Charles Mitchell, president of the National City Bank, the Rockefeller bank, Carl Bosch, Paul Warburg, Herman Schmitz and Schmitz' nephew, Max Ilgner.

Although his name is hardly known, Frank Howard was for many years a key figure in Standard Oil operations as director of its research and its international agreements. He also was chairman of the research committee at Sloan Kettering Institute during the 1930s; his appointee at Sloan Kettering, Dusty Rhoads, headed the experimentation in the development of chemotherapy. During the Second World War, Rhoads headed the Chemical Warfare Service in Washington at U.S. Army Headquarters. It was Frank Howard who had persuaded both Alfred Sloan and Charles Kettering of General Motors in 1939 to give their fortunes to the Cancer Center, which then took on their names. A member of the wealthy Atherton family, Frank Howard (1890-1964) had married a second time, his second wife being a leading member of the British aristocracy, the Duchess of Leeds. The first Duke of Leeds was titled in 1694, Sir Thomas Osborne, who was one of the key conspirators in the overthrow of King James II and the seizure of the throne of England by William III in 1688. Osborne had made peace with Holland during the reign of King Charles II, and singlehandedly promoted the marriage of Mary, daughter of the Duke of York, to William of Orange in 1677. The Dictionary of National Biography notes that Osborne "for five years managed the House of Commons by corruption and enriched himself." He was impeached by King Charles II for treasonous negotiations with King Louis XIV and imprisoned in the Tower of London from 1678 to 1684. After his release, he again became active in the conspiracy to bring in William of Orange as King of England and secured the crucial province of York for him. William then created him Duke of Leeds. The placing of William on the throne of England made it possible for the conspirators to implement the crucial step in their plans, setting up the Bank of England in 1694. This enabled the Amsterdam bankers to gain control of the wealth of the British Empire. Osborne's biography also notes that he was later accused of Jacobinite intrigues and was impeached for receiving a large bribe to procure the charter for the East India Company in 1695, but "the proceedings were not concluded." It was further noted that he "left a large fortune."

The 11th Duke of Leeds was Minister to Washington from 1931 to 1935, Minister to the Holy See from 1936 to 1947, that is, throughout the Second World War. One branch of the family married into the Delano family, becoming relatives of Franklin Delano Roosevelt. A cousin, Viscount Chandos, was a prominent British official, serving in the War Cabinet under Churchill from 1942 to 1945, later becoming a director of the Rothschild firm, Alliance Assurance, and Imperial Chemical Industries.

Frank Howard was the key official in maintaining relations between Standard Oil and I. G. Farben. He led in the development of synthetic rubber, which was crucial to

Germany in the Second World War; he later wrote a book,'
'Buna Rubber." He also was the consultant to the drug firm,
Rohm and Haas, representing the Rockefeller connection
with that firm. In his later years, he resided in Paris, but
continued to maintain his office at 30 Rockefeller Center,
New York.

Walter Teagle, the president of Standard Oil, owned
500,000 shares of American I. G., these shares later
becoming the basis of the Teagle Foundation. Herman
Metz, who was also a director of American I. G., was
president of H. A. Metz Company, New York, a drug firm
wholly owned by I. G. Farben of Germany. Francis Garvan,
who had served as Alien Property Custodian during the First
World War, knew many secrets of I. G. Farben's operations.
He was prosecuted in 1929 to force him to remain silent.
The action was brought by the Department of Justice
through Attorney General Merton Lewis, the former counsel
for Bosch Company. John Krim, former counsel for the
German Embassy in the United States, testified that Senator
John King had been on the payroll of the Hamburg
American Line for three years at a salary of fifteen thousand
dollars a year; he appointed Otto Kahn as treasurer of his
election fund. Homer Cummings, who had been Attorney
General for six years, then became counsel for General
Aniline and Film at a salary of $100,000 a year. During the
Second World War, GAF was supposedly owned by a Swiss
firm; it came under considerable suspicion as an "enemy"
concern and was finally taken over by the United States
government. John Foster Dulles had been director of GAF
from 1927 to 1934; he was also a director of International
Nickel, which was part of the network of I. G. Farben firms.
Dulles was related to the Rockefeller family through the
Avery connection. He was attorney for the organization of a
new investment firm, set up by Avery Rockefeller, in 1936
which was called Schroder- Rockefeller Company. It
combined operations of the Schroder Bank, Hitler's

personal bank and the Rockefeller interests. Baron Kurt van Schroder was one of Hitler's closest confidantes, and a leading officer of the SS. He was head of the Keppler Associates, which funnelled money to the SS for leading German Corporations. Keppler was the official in charge of Industrial Fats during Goering's Four Year Plan, which was launched in 1936.

American I. G. changed its name to General Aniline and Film during the Second World War, but it was still wholly owned by I. G. Chemie of Switzerland, a subsidiary of I. G. Farben of Germany. It was headed by Gadow, brother-in-law of Herman Schmitz. I. G. Farben's international agreements directly affected the U.S. war effort, because they set limits on U.S. supplies of magnesium, synthetic rubber and crucial medical supplies. The director of I. G Farben's dyestuffs division, Baron George von Schnitzler, was related to the powerful von Rath family, the J. H. Stein Bankhaus which held Hitler's account and the von Mallinckrodt family, the founders of the drug firm in the United States. Like other I. G. officials, he had become an enthusiastic supporter of the Hitler regime. I. G. Farben gave four and a half million Reichsmarks to the Nazi Party in 1933; by 1945, I. G. had given the Party 40 million reichsmarks, a sum which equalled all contributions by I. G. to all other recipients during that period. One scholar of the Nazi era, Anthony Sutton, has focussed heavily on German supporters of Hitler, while ignoring the crucial role played by the Bank of England and its Governor, Sir Montague Norman, in financing the Nazi regime. Sutton's position on this problem may have been influenced by the fact that he is British. In view of the outspoken statements from Adolf Hitler about Jewish influence in Germany, it would be difficult to explain the role of I. G. Farben in the Nazi era. Peter Hayes' definitive study of I. G. Farben shows that in 1933, it had ten Jews on its governing boards. We have previously pointed out that I. G., from its inception was a

Rothschild concern, formulated by the House of Rothschild and implemented through its agents, Max Warburg in Germany and Standard Oil in the United States.

Prince Bernhard of the Netherlands joined the SS during the early 1930s. He then joined the board of an I. G. subsidiary, Farben Bilder, from which he took the name of his postwar supersecret policy making group, the Bilderbergers. Farben executives played an important role in organizing the Circle of Friends for Heinrich Himmler, although it was initially known as Keppler's Circle of Friends, Keppler being the chairman of an I. G. subsidiary. His nephew, Fritz J. Kranefuss, was the personal assistant to Heinrich Himmler. Of the forty members of the Circle of Friends, which provided ample funds for Himmler, eight were executives of I. G. Farben or of its subsidiaries.

Despite the incredible devastation of most German cities from World War II air bombings, the I. G. Farben building in Frankfort, one of the largest buildings there, miraculously survived intact. A large Rockefeller mansion in Frankfort also was left untouched by the war, despite the saturation bombing. Frankfort was the birthplace of the Rothschild family. It was hardly coincidental that the postwar government of Germany, Allied Military Government, should set up its offices in the magnificent I. G. Farben building. This government was headed by General Lucius Clay, who later became a partner of Lehmen Brothers bankers in New York. The Political Division was headed by Robert Murphy, who would preside at the Nuremberg Trials, where he was successful in glossing over the implication of I. G. Farben officials and Baron Kurt von Schroder. Schroder was held a short time in a detention camp and then set free to return to his banking business. The Economic Division was headed by Lewis Douglas, son of the founder of Memorial Cancer center in New York, president of Mutual Life and director of General Motors.

Douglas was slated to become U.S. High Commissioner for Germany, but he agreed to step aside in favor of his brother-in-law, John J. McCloy. By an interesting circumstance, Douglas, McCloy and Chancellor Konrad Adenauer of Germany had all married sisters, the daughters of John Zinsser, a partner of J. P. Morgan Company.

As the world's pre-eminent cartel, I. G. Farben and the drug companies which it controlled in the United States through the Rockefeller interests were responsible for many inexplicable developments in the production and distribution of drugs. From 1908 to 1936, I. G. held back its discovery of sulfanilimide, which would become a potent weapon in the medical arsenal. In 1920, I. G. had signed working agreements with the important drug firms of Switzerland, Sandoz and Ciba-Geigy. In 1926, I. G. merged with Dynamit-Nobel, the German branch of the dynamite firm, while an English firm took over the English division. I. G. officials then began to negotiate with Standard Oil officials about the prospective manufacture of synthetic coal, which would present a serious threat to Standard Oil's monopoly. A compromise was reached with the establishment of American I. G., in which both firms would play an active role and share in the profits.

Charles Higham's book,"Trading with the Enemy," offers ample documentation of the Rockefeller activities during the Second World War. While Hitler's bombers were dropping tons of explosives on London, they were paying royalties on every gallon of gasoline they burned to Standard Oil, under existing patent agreements. After World War II, when Queen Elizabeth visited the United States, she stayed in only one private home during her visit, the Kentucky estate of William Farish, of Standard Oil. Nelson Rockefeller moved to Washington after our involvement in World War II, where Roosevelt named him Coordinator of Inter-American Affairs. Apparently his principal task was to coordinate the refueling of German ships in South America from Standard Oil tanks. He also used this office to obtain important South American concessions for his private firm, International Basic Exonomy Corporation, including a corner on the Colombian coffee market. He promptly upped the price, a move which enabled him to buy seven billion dollars worth of real estate in South America and also gave rise to the stereotype of the "Yanqui imperialismo." The attack on Vice President Nixon's automobile when he visited South America was explained by American officials as a direct result of the depredations of the Rockefellers, which caused widespread agitation against Americans in Latin America.

After World War II, twenty-four German executives were prosecuted by the victors, all of them connected with I. G. Farben, including eleven officers of I. G. Eight were acquitted, including Max Ilgner, nephew of Harman Schmitz. Schmitz received the most severe sentence, eight years. Ilgner actually received three years, but the time was credited against his time in jail waiting for trial, and he was immediately released. The Judge was C. G. Shake and the prosecuting attorney was Al Minskoff.

The survival of I. G. Farben was headlined by the Wall Street Journal on May 3,1988—GERMANY BEATS WORLD IN CHEMICAL SALES. Reporter Thomas F. O'Boyle listed the world's top five chemical companies in 1987 as 1. BASF $25.8 billion dollars 2. Bayer $23.6 billion dollars. 3. Hoechst $23.5 billion dollars. 4. ICI $20 billion dollars. 5. DuPont $17 billion dollars in chemical sales only.

The first three companies are the firms resulting from the "dismantling" of I. G. Farben from 1945 to 1952 by the Allied Military Government, in a process suspiciously similar to the "dismantling" of the Standard Oil empire by court edict in 1911. The total sales computed in dollars of the three spin-offs of I. G. Farben, some $72 billion, dwarfs its nearest rivals, ICI and DuPont, who together amount to about half of the Farben empire's dollar sales in 1987. Hoechst bought Celanese corp. in 1987 for $2.72 billion.

O'Boyle notes that "The Big Three (Farben spinoffs) still behave like a cartel. Each dominates specific areas; head to head competition is limited. Critics suspect collusion. At the least, there's a coziness that doesn't exist in the U.S. chemical industry."

After the war, Americans were told they must support an "altruistic" plan to rebuild devastated Europe, to be called the Marshall Plan, after Chief of Staff George Marshall, who had been labelled on the floor of the Senate by Senator Joseph McCarthy as "a living lie." The Marshall Plan proved to be merely another Rockefeller Plan to loot the American taxpayer. On December 13, 1948, Col. Robert McCormick, editor of the *Chicago Tribune,* personally denounced Esso's looting of the Marshall Plan in a signed editorial. The Marshall Plan had been rushed through Congress by a powerful and vocal group, headed by Winthrop Aldrich, president of the Chase Manhattan Bank and Nelson Rockefeller's brother-in-law, ably seconded by Nelson Rockefeller and William Clayton, the head of Anderson, Clayton Company. The Marshall Plan proved to be but one of a number of lucrative postwar swindles, which included the Bretton Woods Agreement, United Nations Relief and Rehabilitation and others.

After World War II, the Rockefellers used their war profits to buy a large share of Union Miniere du Haut Katanga, and African copper lode owned by Belgian interest, including the Societe Generale, a Jesuit controlled bank. Soon after their investment, the Rockefellers launched a bold attempt to seize total control of the mines through sponsoring a local revolution, using as their agent the

Grangesberg operation. This enterprise had originally been developed by Sir Ernest Cassel, financial advisor to King Edward VII—Cassel's daughter later married Lord Mountbatten, a member of the British royal family, who was also related to the Rothschilds. Grangesberg was now headed by Bo Hammarskjold, whose brother, Dag Hammarskjold was then Secretary General of the United Nations—Bo Hammarskjold became a casualty of the Rockefeller revolution when his plane was shot down during hostilities in the Congo. Various stories have since circulated about who killed him and why he was killed. The Rockefeller intervention in the Congo was carried out by their able lieutenants, Dean Rusk and George Ball of the State Department and by Fowler Hamilton.

In the United States, the Rockefeller interests continue to play the major political role. Old John D. Rockefeller's treasurer at Standard Oil, Charles Pratt, bequeathed his New York mansion to the Council on Foreign Relations as its world headquarters. His grandson, George Pratt Shultz, is now Secretary of State. The Rockefellers also wielded a crucial role through their financing of the Trotskyite Communist group in the United States, the League for Industrial Democracy, whose directors include such staunch "anti- Communists" as Jeane Kirkpatrick and Sidney Hook. The Rockefellers were also active on the "rightwing" front through their sponsorship of the John Birch Society. To enable Robert Welch, a 32nd degree Mason, to devote all of his time to the John Birch Society, Nelson Rockefeller purchased his family firm, the Welch Candy Company, from him at a handsome price. Welch chose the principal officers of the John Birch Society from his acquaintances at the Council On Foreign Relations. For years afterwards, American patriots were puzzled by the consistent inability of the John Birch Society to move forward on any of its well-advertised "anti-Communist" goals. The fact that the society had been set up at the behest of the backers of the world

Communist revolution may have played some role in this development. Other patriots wondered why most American conservative writers, including the present writer, were steadily blacklisted by the John Birch Society for some thirty years. Despite thousands of requests from would be book buyers, the John Birch Society refused to review or list any of my books. After several decades of futility, the Society was totally discredited by its own record. In a desperate effort to restore its image, William Buckley, the CIA propagandist, launched a "fierce" attack against the John Birch Society in the pages of his magazine, the *National Review*. This free publicity campaign also did little to revive the moribund organization.

The Rockefeller monopoly influence has had its effect on some of New York's largest and wealthiest churches. Trinity Church on Wall Street, whose financial resources had been directed by none other than J. P. Morgan, owns some forty commercial properties in Manhattan and has a stock portfolio of $50 million, which, due to informed investment, actually yields a return of $25 million a year! Only $2.6 million of this income is spent for charitable work. The rector, who receives a salary of $100,000 a year, lives on the fashionable Upper East Side. Trinity's mausoleum sells its spaces at fees started at $1250 and rising to $20,000. St. Bartholomews, on Fifth Avenue, has an annual budget of $3.2 million a year of which only $100,000 is spent on charity. Its rector resides in a thirteen room apartment on Park Avenue.

In medicine, the Rockefeller influence remains entrenched in its Medical Monopoly. We have mentioned its control of the cancer industry through the Sloan Kettering Cancer Center. We have listed the directors of the major drug firms, each with its director from Chase Manhattan Bank, the Standard Oil Company or other Rockefeller firms. The American College of Surgeons maintains a monopolistic control of hospitals through the powerful Hospital Survey Committee, with members Winthrop Aldrich and David McAlpine Pyle representing the Rockefeller control.

A medical fraternity known as the "rich man's club," the New York Academy of Medicine, was offered grants for a new building by the Rockefeller Foundation and the Carnegie Foundation, its subsidiary group. This "seed money" was then used to finance a public campaign which brought in funds to erect a new building. For Director of the new facility, the Rockefellers chose Dr. Lindsly Williams, son-in-law of the managing partner of Kidder, Peabody, a firm strongly affiliated with the J. P. Morgan interests (the J. P. Morgan Company had originally been called the Peabody Company). Williams was married to Grace Kidder Ford. Although Dr. Williams was widely known to be an incompetent physician, his family connections were impeccable. He became a factor in Franklin D. Roosevelt's election campaign when he publicly certified that Roosevelt, a cripple in a wheelchair who suffered from a number of oppressive ailments, was both physically and mentally fit to be the President of United States. Dr. Williams' opinion, published in an article in the widely circulated *Collier's Magazine,"* allayed public doubts about Roosevelt's condition. As a result, Williams was to be offered a newly created post in Roosevelt's cabinet, Secretary of Health. However, it was another thirty years before Health became a cabinet post, due to the politicking of Oscar Ewing.

The Rockefellers had greatly extended their business interests in the impoverished Southern states by establishing the Rockefeller Sanitary Commission. It was headed by Dr. Wickliffe Rose, a longtime Rockefeller henchman whose name appears on the original charter of the Rockefeller Foundation. Despite its philanthropic goals, the Rockefeller Sanitary Commission required financial contributions from each of the eleven Southern states in which it operated, resulting in the creation of State Departments of Health in those states and opening up important new spheres of influence for their Drug Trust. In Tennessee, the Rockefeller representative was a Dr. Olin West, who moved on to Chicago to become the power behind the scenes at the American Medical Association for forty years, as secretary and general manager.

The Rockefeller Institute for Medical Research finally dropped the "Medical Research" part of its title; its president, Dr. Detlev Bronk, resided in a $600,000 mansion furnished by this charitable operation. Rockefeller's general Education Board has spent more than $100 million to gain control of the nation's medical schools and turn our physicians to physicians of the allopathic school, dedicated to surgery and the heavy use of drugs. The Board, which had developed from the original Peabody Foundation, also spent some $66 million for Negro education.

One of the most far-reaching consequences of the General Education Board's political philosophy was achieved with a mere six million dollar grant to Columbia University in 1917, to set up the "progressive" Lincoln School. From this school descended the national network of progressive educators and social scientists, whose pernicious influence closely paralleled the goals of the Communist Party, another favorite recipient of the Rockefeller millions. From its outset, the Lincoln School was described frankly as a revolutionary school for the primary and secondary schools of the entire United States. It immediately discarded all theories of education which were based on formal and well-established disciplines, that is, the McGuffey Reader type of education which worked by teaching such subjects as Latin and algebra, thus teaching children to think logically about problems. Rockefeller biographer Jules Abel hails the Lincoln School as "a beacon light in progressive education."

Rockefeller Institute financial fellowships produced many prominent workers in our atomic programs, such as J. Robert Oppenheimer, who was later removed from government laboratories as a suspected Soviet agent. Although most of his friends and associates were known Soviet agents, this was called "guilt by association." The Rockefeller Foundation created a number of spinoff groups, which now plague the nation with a host of ills, one of them being the Social Science Research Council, which single-handedly spawned the nationwide "poverty industry," a business which expends some $130 billion a year of taxpayer funds while grossing some $6 billion income for its practitioners. The money, which would amply feed and house all of the nation's "poor," is dissipated through a vast administrative network which awards generous concessions to a host of parasitic "consultants."

Despite years of research, the present writer has been able to merely scratch the surface of the Rockefeller influences listed here. For instance, the huge Burroughs Wellcome drug firm is wholly owned by the "charitable" Wellcome Trust. This trust is directed by Lord Oliver Franks, a key member of the London Connection which maintains the United States as a British Colony. Franks was Ambassador to the United States from 1948 to 1952. He is now a director of the Rockefeller Foundation, as its principal representative in England. He also is a director of the Schroder Bank, which handled Hitler's personal bank account, director of the Rhodes Trust in charge of approving Rhodes scholarships, visiting professor at the University of Chicago and chairman of Lloyd's Bank, one of England's Big Five.

Other Rockefeller Foundation spinoffs include the influential Washington thinktank, the Brookings Institution, the National Bureau of Economic Research, whose findings play a critical role in manipulating the stock market; the

Public Administration Clearing House, which indoctrinates the nation's municipal employees; the Council of State Governments, which controls the nation's state legislatures; and the Institute of Pacific Relations, the most notorious Communist front in the United States. The Rockefellers appeared as directors of this group, funnelling money to it through their financial advisor, Lewis Lichtenstein Strauss, of Kuhn, Loeb Company.

The Rockefellers have maintained their controlling interest in the Chase Manhattan Bank, owning five per cent of the stock. One per cent is generally considered to give working control of a bank. Through this one asset, they control $42.5 billion worth of assets. Chase Manhattan interlocks closely with the Big Four insurance companies, of which three, Metropolitan, Equitable and New York Life had $113 billion in assets in 1969.

With the advent of the Reagan Administration in 1980, the Rockefeller interests sought to obscure their longtime support of world Communism, by bringing to Washington a vocally "anti- Communist" administration. Reagan was soon wining and dining Soviet premiers as enthusiastically as had his predecessor Jimmy Carter. The Reagan campaign had been managed by two officials of Bechtel Corporation, its president, George Pratt Schultz, a Standard Oil heir, and his counsel, Casper Weinberger. Shultz was named Secretary of State, Weinberger, Secretary of Defense, Bechtel had been financed by the Schroder-Rockefeller Company, the 1936 alliance between the Schroder Bank and the Rockefeller heirs.

The Rockefeller influence also remains preeminent in the monetary field. Since November, 1910, when Senator Nelson Aldrich chaired the secret conference at Jekyl Island which gave us the Federal Reserve Act, the Rockefellers have kept us within the sphere of the London Connection.

During the Carter Administration, David Rockefeller generously sent his personal assistant, Paul Volcker, to Washington to head the Federal Reserve Board. Reagan finally replaced him in 1987 with Alan Greenspan, a partner of J. P. Morgan Company. Their influence on our banking system has remained constant through many financial coups on their part, one of the most profitable being the confiscation of privately owned gold from American citizens by Roosevelt's edict. Our citizens had to turn over their gold to the privately Federal Reserve System. The Constitution permits confiscation for purposes of eminent domain, but prohibits confiscation for private gain. The gold's new owners then had the gold revalued from $20 an ounce to $35, giving them an enormous profit.

In reviewing the all-pervasive influence of the Rockefellers and their foreign controllers, the Rothschilds, in every aspect of American life, the citizen must ask himself, "What can be done?" Right can prevail only when the citizen actively seeks justice.

Justice can prevail only when each citizen realizes that it is his God- given duty to mete out justice. History has documented all of the crimes of the usurpers of our Constitution. We have learned the painful lession that the Rockefeller monopolists exercise their evil power almost solely through federal and state agents. At this writing, former Congressman Ron Paul is running for the Presidency of the United States on an eminently sensible and practical campaign—abolish the Federal Reserve System—abolish the FBI—abolish the Internal Revenue Service—and abolish the CIA. It has been known for years that 90% of the Federal Bureau of Investigation, ostensibly set up to "fight crime" has been to harass and isolate political dissidents, (including the present writer, over a period of some thirty-three years).

The criminal syndicalists are now looting the American nation of one trillion dollars each year, of which about one-third, more than three hundred billion dollars per year, represents the profitable depredations of the Drug Trust and its medical subsidiaries. Before a sustained effort to combat these depredations can be mounted, Americans must make every effort to regain their health. As Ezra Pound demanded in one of his famous radio broadcasts, "Health, dammit!" America became the greatest and most productive nation in the world because we had the healthiest citizens in the world.

When the Rockefeller Syndicate began its takeover of our medical profession in 1910, our citizens went into a sharp decline. Today, we suffer from a host of debilitating ailments, both mental and physical, nearly all of which can be traced directly to the operations of the chemical and drug monopoly, and which pose the greatest threat to our continued existence as a nation. Unite now to restore our national health—the result will be the restoration of our national pride, the resumption of our role as the inventors and producers of the modern world, and the custodian of the world's hopes and dreams of liberty and freedom.

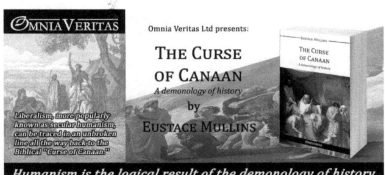
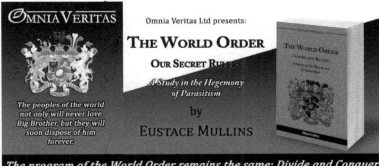
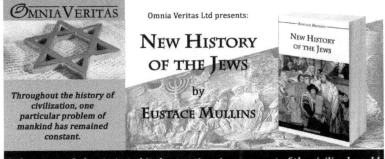
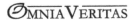

CPSIA information can be obtained
at www.ICGtesting.com
Printed in the USA
BVHW080113280821
615431BV00003BA/85